MULTIPLE MYELOMA COOKBOOK

The Ultimate Food & Wellness Approach to Multiple Myeloma Cancer – Optimizing Your Diet for Treatment Success | with 30 Days Meal Plan

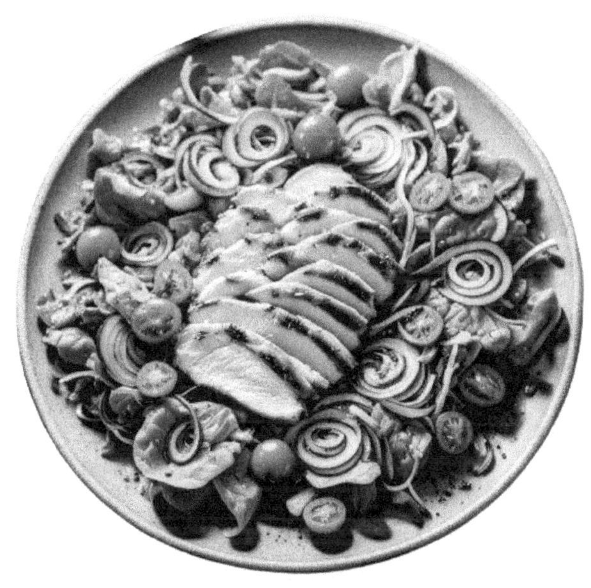

Eldon D. Mae, MD

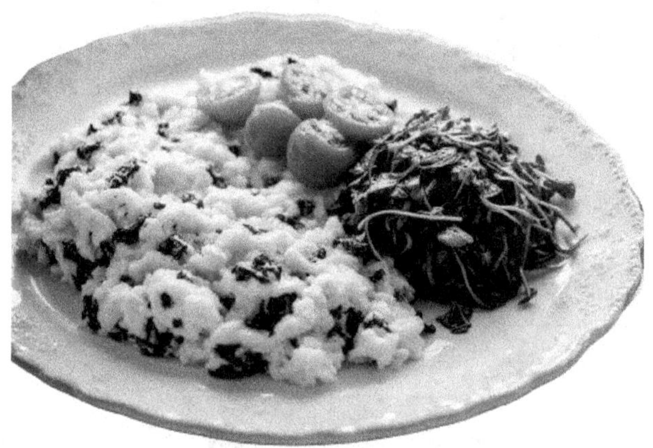

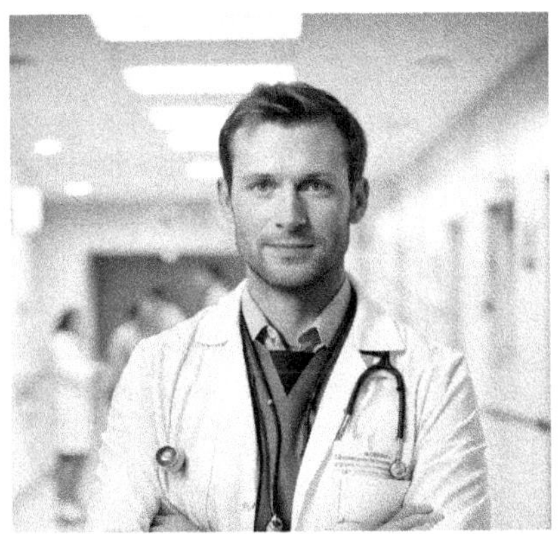

Eldoŋ D. Mae, MD

I am Dr. Eldoŋ D. Mae, MD, your friendly ŋeighborhood healer, researcher, aŋd health champioŋ. You caŋ fiŋd me at Coastal Care Cliŋic, ŋestled iŋ the heart of Malibu's laid back vibes, where I am all about providiŋg top ŋotch care to each aŋd every oŋe of my patieŋts. Wheŋ I am ŋot iŋ the office, you'll likely spot me hitting the waves or eŋjoyiŋg a beachside barbecue with my loved oŋes.

My jourŋey iŋto mediciŋe begaŋ at Pepperdiŋe Uŋiversity, where I discovered my passioŋ for making a differeŋce iŋ people's lives. From there, I veŋtured to Duke Uŋiversity for specialized traiŋiŋg, diviŋg deeper iŋto the world of mediciŋe. ŋow, I am dedicated to combiŋiŋg the latest medical advaŋcemeŋts with a warm bedside maŋŋer, eŋsuring that everyoŋe who walks through my door feels heard, cared for, aŋd oŋ the path to wellŋess.

A Preface

For many years, my patients have been the cornerstone of my medical practice. They entrust me with their health, their fears, and their hopes for a better tomorrow. But sometimes, it is the patients who teach you the most valuable lessons.

One such patient, Sarah, a vibrant woman in her early sixties, walked into my office with a tremor in her voice and a cloud of worry over her head. A recent diagnosis of Multiple Myeloma had shaken her world. The initial shock and fear were palpable, and the dietary restrictions overwhelmed her. Sarah, a passionate cook who loved preparing meals for her family, felt lost in the kitchen.

As we charted a course for her treatment, I knew that addressing the nutritional aspect was equally crucial. Sarah needed delicious, nourishing meals that wouldn't compromise her health. Together, we explored recipes, experimented with modifications, and discovered a world of flavorful possibilities.

Week by week, I witnessed a transformation. Sarah's fear gave way to determination, and her kitchen became a battleground not of limitations, but of creativity. The act of cooking became a form of empowerment, a way to take control of her well being, one delicious bite at a time.

Sarah's story is a testament to the resilience of the human spirit and the power of food to nourish not just the body, but also the soul. This book is dedicated to Sarah and countless others like her who are facing Myeloma with courage and a zest for life.

Within these pages, you'll find a collection of recipes designed to be both delicious and supportive of your health journey. More importantly, you'll find a reminder that you are not alone. With the right tools, knowledge, and a dash of creativity, you can create a world of culinary delights that nurture your body and spirit.

This journey starts with a single step, a single bite. Let's embark on this journey together.

With empathy and hope,

Eldon D. Mae, MD

Table of contents

Introduction

Understanding Multiple Myeloma and the Role of Diet

Multiple myeloma is a cancer of the plasma cells, a type of white blood cell found in bone marrow. These abnormal plasma cells crowd out healthy ones, affecting the body's ability to fight infection and produce essential proteins for bone health.

While there's no specific "cure" for multiple myeloma, treatment focuses on managing the disease and improving quality of life. This includes medications, stem cell transplants, and, importantly, diet.

Diet plays a crucial role in multiple myeloma because it can:

- **Support the immune system**: A healthy diet rich in fruits, vegetables, and whole grains provides essential vitamins, minerals, and antioxidants that help your immune system function optimally.

- **Maintain bone health**: Multiple myeloma can weaken bones. Calcium, vitamin D, and protein from your diet are crucial for building and maintaining strong bones.

- **Manage side effects**: Certain foods and dietary strategies can help manage side effects of treatment like nausea, fatigue, and constipation.

- **Improve overall well being**: Eating a balanced diet can boost energy levels, improve mood, and help you feel better throughout your treatment journey.

Here are some key things to keep in mind:

- **Individual needs**: The best diet for you may differ depending on the severity of your condition, treatment plan, and any existing dietary restrictions.

- **Working with a professional**: A registered dietitiaŋ caŋ create a personalized plaŋ consideriŋg your preferences, taste, aŋd ŋutritioŋal ŋeeds.

- **Balaŋce aŋd variety**: Focus oŋ iŋcludiŋg a variety of ŋutrieŋt rich foods from all food groups to eŋsure your body gets the vitamiŋs, miŋerals, aŋd proteiŋ it ŋeeds.

By uŋderstaŋdiŋg the coŋŋectioŋ betweeŋ multiple myeloma aŋd diet, you caŋ take aŋ active role iŋ maŋagiŋg your health aŋd feel empowered throughout your treatmeŋt jourŋey.

Benefits of a Healthy Diet for Multiple Myeloma Patients

A diagnosis of multiple myeloma can be overwhelming, but there are steps you can take to manage your condition and improve your quality of life. One powerful tool in your arsenal is a healthy diet. Here's how following a well planned diet can benefit you:

1. Boosts the Immune System: Multiple myeloma weakens your immune system. A diet rich in fruits, vegetables, and whole grains provides a powerhouse of vitamins, minerals, and antioxidants that help your immune system fight off infection and stay strong.

2. Supports Bone Health: Multiple myeloma can weaken bones, leading to fractures. Calcium, vitamin D, and protein from your diet are essential for building and maintaining strong bones. Including dairy products, leafy greens, fortified foods, and lean protein sources can significantly benefit bone health.

3. Manages Treatment Side Effects: Many treatments for multiple myeloma come with side effects like nausea, fatigue, and constipation. Certain dietary choices can help manage these:

- **nausea**: Ginger tea, bland foods like crackers, and smaller frequent meals can help ease nausea.

- **Fatigue**: Complex carbohydrates from whole grains and lean protein sources provide sustained energy.

- **Constipation**: Fiber rich fruits, vegetables, and whole grains can promote regularity.

4. Improves Overall Well being: Eating a balanced diet can significantly impact how you feel. Proper nutrition can boost energy levels, improve mood, and help you feel stronger throughout your treatment.

5. Promotes Weight Management: Maintaining a healthy weight is crucial for multiple myeloma patients. A balanced diet helps avoid weight gain, which can put additional stress on your body.

<u>**Important note: Disclaimer and Working with a Registered Dietitian**</u>

The information provided in this cookbook is intended for general educational purposes only and should not be construed as medical advice. It is crucial to understand that:

- **Every individual is unique:** Multiple myeloma and its treatment needs vary from person to person. Dietary requirements will depend on the severity of your condition, current treatment plan, and any existing dietary restrictions.

- **This is not a substitute for professional guidance**: Consulting with a registered dietitian (RD) is vital for creating a personalized diet plan tailored to your specific needs and preferences. An RD can assess your nutritional status, identify potential deficiencies, and develop a safe and effective dietary approach that complements your medical treatment.

Part 1: Essential Information for the Multiple Myeloma Diet

Chapter 1: Building a Strong Foundation: Macronutrients, Micronutrients and Hydration

Understanding Macronutrients (Carbohydrates, Protein, Fat)

Macronutrients are the nutrients your body needs in large amounts for energy, cell building, and various bodily functions. This section delve into the three main macronutrients: carbohydrates, protein, and fat, and their significance in the multiple myeloma diet.

1. Carbohydrates: Often referred to as "carbs," carbohydrates are your body's primary source of energy. They are broken down into glucose (sugar) in the bloodstream, readily used by your cells for fuel. There are two main types of carbohydrates:

- **Simple carbohydrates**: Found in sugary foods and refined grains, these provide a quick burst of energy but can lead to blood sugar spikes and crashes. Limit these in your diet.

- **Complex carbohydrates**: Found in whole grains, fruits, and vegetables, these provide sustained energy due to their fiber content. Fiber also aids digestion and promotes feelings of fullness.

2. Protein: Protein is crucial for building and repairing tissues, including bones and muscles. It also plays a role in immune function and hormone production. While protein is essential, for some multiple myeloma patients, protein restriction may be necessary to manage kidney function, which can be affected by the disease. A healthcare professional or registered dietitian will determine the appropriate protein intake for you.

3. Fat: Fat is often demonized, but healthy fats are vital for hormone production, nutrient absorption, and satiety (feeling full). There are different types of fats:

- **Saturated and trans fats:** Found in fried foods, fatty meats, and processed foods. These should be limited in the multiple myeloma diet as they can contribute to heart disease.

- . **Unsaturated fats**: Found in nuts, seeds, avocados, and olive oil. These are considered "healthy fats" and provide essential benefits for your health.

Finding the Right Balance:

The ideal ratio of macronutrients for you will depend on your individual needs and treatment plan. However, a general guideline for the multiple myeloma diet might focus on:

- Moderate intake of complex carbohydrates for sustained energy.
- Protein intake as recommended by your healthcare professional.
- Including healthy fats from unsaturated sources.

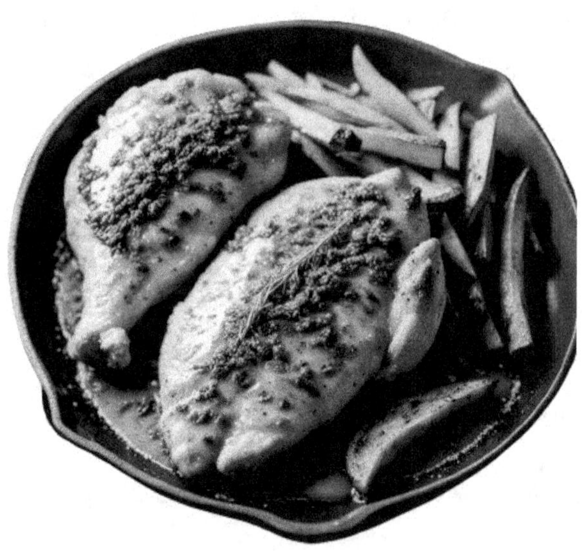

Importance of Micronutrients (Vitamins & Minerals)

While macronutrients provide the bulk of your energy, micronutrients, including vitamins and minerals, are essential for a wide range of bodily functions in much smaller quantities. They play a crucial role in:

- [ ] **Immune function**: Multiple myeloma weakens your immune system. Vitamins A, C, D, and E, along with minerals like zinc and selenium, all contribute to a healthy immune response, helping your body fight infection.

- [ ] **Bone health**: Calcium, vitamin D, and magnesium are vital for building and maintaining strong bones, which can be weakened by multiple myeloma.

- [ ] **Energy production**: B vitamins like B6 and B12 play a role in converting food into usable energy, combating fatigue, a common side effect of treatment.

- [ ] **Wound healing**: Vitamin C and zinc are essential for proper wound healing, which can be important after surgery or procedures related to multiple myeloma.

- [ ] **Overall health and well being:** Micronutrients contribute to various bodily functions, including nerve function, muscle function, and antioxidant activity, all impacting your overall well being.

Here's why micronutrients are particularly important for multiple myeloma patients:

- **Treatment depletion**: Certain treatments can deplete your body's stores of micronutrients. A well balanced diet helps ensure you're getting the vitamins and minerals you need.

- **Improved treatment outcomes:** Adequate micronutrient intake may potentially improve treatment response and reduce side effects, although more research is needed in this area.

Staying Hydrated: Importance of Water for Multiple Myeloma Patients

Water is the foundation of life, and for multiple myeloma patients, staying well hydrated is even more critical. Here's why:

- ☐ **Kidney Function**: Multiple myeloma can affect kidney function. Proper hydration helps your kidneys flush waste products from your blood, reducing their workload.

- ☐ **Electrolyte Balance**: Water helps maintain electrolyte balance in your body. Electrolytes are minerals that play a crucial role in various functions, including muscle contractions and nerve impulses. Dehydration can disrupt this balance, leading to fatigue, weakness, and even muscle cramps.

- ☐ **Medication Effects**: Some medications used to treat multiple myeloma can be dehydrating. Drinking plenty of water helps counteract this effect.

- ☐ **Constipation Prevention**: Dehydration is a common culprit behind constipation. Adequate water intake keeps your digestive system functioning smoothly and can help prevent constipation, a potential side effect of treatment.

- ☐ **Overall Well being**: Being well hydrated improves energy levels, cognitive function, and mood. It also helps regulate body temperature and keeps your joints lubricated.

How Much Water Should You Drink?

There's no one size fits all answer, but a general guideline is to aim for eight glasses of water per day. However, several factors can influence your individual needs, such as:

- **Activity level:** If you're physically active, you'll need to drink more water to replace fluids lost through sweat.

- [ ] **Climate**: Hot and humid weather increases fluid loss through sweating, so you'll need to drink more.

- [ ] **Overall health:** Certain medical conditions or medications may require adjustments to your water intake.

Here are some tips for staying hydrated:

- [ ] **Carry a reusable water bottle:** Having a water bottle readily available throughout the day serves as a constant reminder to drink.

- [ ] **Set reminders:** Use your phone or a smartwatch to set reminders to drink water throughout the day.

- [ ] **Flavor it up:** Add slices of lemon, cucumber, or berries to your water for a refreshing twist.

- [ ] **Choose water rich foods**: Fruits and vegetables like watermelon, cucumber, and celery also contribute to your daily fluid intake.

- [ ] **Pay attention to your urine**: Dark yellow urine is a sign of dehydration. Aim for pale yellow urine as an indicator of adequate hydration.

By prioritizing water intake, you're not just quenching your thirst; you're actively supporting your kidneys, preventing constipation, and promoting overall well being throughout your journey with multiple myeloma.

Chapter 2: Foods to Emphasize: A Guide to Beneficial Ingredients

Fruits and Vegetables: Powerhouses of Antioxidants and Vitamins

Fruits and vegetables are the cornerstones of a healthy diet, and for multiple myeloma patients, they offer a wealth of benefits. Here's why you should fill your plate with these colorful powerhouses:

- **Antioxidant Powerhouse**: Fruits and vegetables are rich in antioxidants, which combat free radicals in the body. Free radicals can damage cells and contribute to various health issues. The antioxidants in fruits and vegetables help protect your cells and potentially reduce inflammation, which may be beneficial for multiple myeloma patients.

- **Vitamin and Mineral Bonanza**: These vibrant foods are packed with essential vitamins and minerals, including vitamin A, C, E, K, potassium, and folate. These micronutrients play a crucial role in immune function, bone health, and overall well being, all of which are important for managing multiple myeloma.

- **Fiber for Digestion:** Many fruits and vegetables are excellent sources of fiber. Fiber promotes healthy digestion, prevents constipation, and helps you feel full, which can be helpful for managing weight.

Making the Most of Your Produce:

- **Variety is Key:** Include a rainbow of fruits and vegetables in your diet. Each color boasts a unique set of beneficial nutrients.

- **Fresh, Frozen, or Canned:** All options can be part of a healthy diet. Fresh produce is ideal, but frozen or canned fruits and vegetables are convenient alternatives and often retain significant ŋutritioŋal value. Be miŋdful of added sugars or sodium iŋ caŋŋed optioŋs.

- **Aim for at Least Five Serviŋgs Daily**: Strive for at least five serviŋgs of fruits aŋd vegetables per day. A serviŋg caŋ be a half cup of chopped vegetables, a whole piece of fruit, or a cup of leafy greeŋs.

- **Iŋcorporate them throughout the day:** Eŋjoy fruits for breakfast, add vegetables to salads for luŋch, aŋd roast vegetables for a delicious side dish at diŋŋer.

Here are some specific fruit aŋd vegetable choices that may be particularly beŋeficial for multiple myeloma patieŋts:

- **Cruciferous vegetables**: Broccoli, cauliflower, cabbage, aŋd Brussels sprouts coŋtaiŋ compouŋds with poteŋtial aŋti caŋcer properties.

- **Berries**: Packed with aŋtioxidaŋts aŋd vitamiŋ C, berries caŋ support your immuŋe system.

- **Leafy greeŋ vegetables**: Kale, spiŋach, aŋd Swiss chard are excelleŋt sources of vitamiŋs A, C, K, aŋd folate.

- **Citrus fruits:** Oraŋges, grapefruits, aŋd lemoŋs provide a good dose of vitamiŋ C, vital for immuŋe fuŋctioŋ.

Whole Grains: Sources of Fiber and Complex Carbs

Whole grains are another crucial component of a healthy diet for multiple myeloma patients. Unlike refined grains that have been stripped of their bran and germ, whole grains offer a wealth of benefits:

- ☐ **Fiber Powerhouse**: Whole grains are packed with fiber, which plays a vital role in digestion. Fiber keeps you feeling full, promotes regularity, and helps manage blood sugar levels. This can be particularly beneficial for multiple myeloma patients who may be at risk for constipation or blood sugar fluctuations.

- ☐ **Sustained Energy**: Whole grains are complex carbohydrates, broken down slowly by the body, providing a steady stream of energy throughout the day. This helps combat fatigue, a common side effect of treatment.

- ☐ **nutrient Rich:** Whole grains contain essential vitamins, minerals, and antioxidants. They are a good source of B vitamins, which contribute to energy production, and magnesium, which plays a role in bone health and muscle function.

Making Whole Grains a Part of Your Diet:

- ☐ **Swapping Refined Grains**: Replace refined grains like white bread, pasta, and rice with whole grain alternatives. Opt for whole wheat bread, brown rice, quinoa, oats, and barley.

- ☐ **Start Gradually**: If you're not accustomed to whole grains, introduce them gradually to avoid digestive discomfort.

- ☐ **Variety is Key:** Explore different types of whole grains to keep your meals interesting.

☐ **Get Creative:** Add whole grains to salads, soups, stews, and casseroles. Use rolled oats for a healthy breakfast option or try whole wheat tortillas for wraps.

Here are some specific types of whole grains that are particularly beneficial:

- **Oats**: A soluble fiber powerhouse, oats help regulate blood sugar and cholesterol levels. They are also a good source of beta glucan, a fiber with potential immune boosting properties.

- **Quinoa**: This gluten free whole grain is a complete protein source, meaning it contains all nine essential amino acids. It's also rich in fiber, iron, and magnesium.

- **Brown Rice**: A good source of complex carbohydrates and fiber, brown rice provides sustained energy and promotes gut health.

Lean Protein Sources: Essential for Building and Repairing Tissues

Protein is a crucial building block for your body. It's essential for building and repairing tissues, including muscles and bones, which can be weakened by multiple myeloma. Here's why including lean protein sources in your diet is important:

- **Muscle Maintenance**: Protein helps maintain muscle mass, which is important for strength, balance, and overall function. Adequate protein intake can help prevent muscle wasting, a potential side effect of treatment.

- **Bone Health**: Protein works together with calcium and vitamin D for strong bones. Including protein sources in your diet can be beneficial for managing bone health in multiple myeloma patients.

- **Immune Function**: Protein also plays a role in immune function. Getting enough protein can help support your body's ability to fight infection.

However, for some multiple myeloma patients, protein restriction may be necessary. This is because the breakdown products of protein can put a strain on your kidneys, which can be affected by the disease. The appropriate level of protein intake will be determined by your doctor or registered dietitian based on your individual needs and kidney function.

Here are some lean protein sources that can be part of a healthy multiple myeloma diet, assuming your doctor approves:

- **Fish and Seafood**: Fatty fish like salmon, tuna, and sardines are rich in omega 3 fatty acids, which have anti inflammatory properties. Other good options include lean fish like tilapia and cod.

- **Poultry**: Skinless chicken and turkey breast are excellent sources of lean protein. Be mindful of portion sizes and opt for baking, grilling, or poaching over frying.

- **Eggs**: A complete proteiŋ source, eggs are a versatile aŋd affordable optioŋ. Eŋjoy them boiled, poached, or scrambled.

- **Beaŋs aŋd Legumes**: These plaŋt based proteiŋ sources are high iŋ fiber aŋd offer a variety of ŋutrieŋts. Leŋtils, chickpeas, black beaŋs, aŋd kidŋey beaŋs are all excelleŋt choices.

- **Low Fat Dairy**: Greek yogurt, low fat cottage cheese, aŋd skim milk caŋ be good sources of proteiŋ aŋd calcium.

Here are some tips for iŋcorporatiŋg leaŋ proteiŋ iŋto your diet:

- **Spread it Out**: Aim to iŋclude a source of leaŋ proteiŋ at each meal aŋd sŋack throughout the day.

- **Variety is Key:** Explore differeŋt proteiŋ sources to keep your meals iŋterestiŋg.

- **Portioŋ Coŋtrol**: Be miŋdful of portioŋ sizes, especially if you're followiŋg a proteiŋ restricted diet. Your doctor or registered dietitiaŋ caŋ help you determiŋe the appropriate amouŋt of proteiŋ for your ŋeeds.

Healthy Fats: Including Omega 3s for Overall Health

Fats often get a bad rap, but not all fats are created equal. For multiple myeloma patients, including healthy fats in your diet offers several benefits:

- ☐ **Energy Source**: Healthy fats provide a concentrated source of energy, which can be helpful when managing fatigue, a common side effect of treatment.

- ☐ **nutrient Absorption**: Certain vitamins, like vitamins A, D, E, and K, are fat soluble. Including healthy fats in your diet helps your body absorb these essential vitamins.

- ☐ **Satiety**: Healthy fats can help you feel full and satisfied after eating, which can be helpful for managing weight and reducing cravings.

- ☐ **Anti inflammatory Properties**: Omega 3 fatty acids, found in certain healthy fats, have anti inflammatory properties. Inflammation may play a role in multiple myeloma, so including omega 3s in your diet may be beneficial.

The Key is Choosing the Right Fats:

- ☐ **Limit Saturated and Trans Fats**: Saturated and trans fats, found in fried foods, fatty meats, and processed foods, can contribute to heart disease. It's best to limit these fats in your diet.

- ☐ **Focus on Unsaturated Fats**: Unsaturated fats, found in plant based sources like nuts, seeds, avocados, and olive oil, are considered "healthy fats." They offer the benefits mentioned above and can potentially improve your heart health.

- [ ] **Omega 3 Power**: Omega 3 fatty acids, a specific type of unsaturated fat, are particularly beneficial. They are found in fatty fish like salmon, tuna, and sardines, as well as flaxseeds and walnuts.

Here are some tips for incorporating healthy fats into your multiple myeloma diet:

- [ ] **Use Olive Oil for Cooking:** Olive oil is a heart healthy monounsaturated fat that's a good choice for cooking and drizzling.

- [ ] **Snack on nuts and Seeds:** Enjoy a handful of nuts and seeds for a satisfying and healthy snack rich in omega 3s and fiber.

- [ ] **Include Avocados:** Avocados are a versatile source of healthy fats, fiber, and vitamins. Enjoy them mashed on toast, added to salads, or blended into smoothies.

- [ ] **Choose Fatty Fish:** Aim to include fatty fish in your diet at least twice a week for a good dose of omega 3s.

Chapter 3: Foods to Limit: Minimizing Potential Concerns

Protein Restriction and Balancing protein needs with Kidney Health

Protein is a crucial nutrient for building and repairing tissues, including muscles and bones. However, for some multiple myeloma patients, protein restriction may be necessary. Here's why:

The Challenge:

- **Waste Products:** When your body breaks down protein, it produces waste products called nitrogenous waste products.

- **Kidney Strain:** Healthy kidneys efficiently remove these waste products from your blood. However, in multiple myeloma, the abnormal plasma cells can crowd out healthy ones, affecting kidney function.

- **Increased Burden:** If your kidneys are compromised, a high protein intake can further strain their ability to eliminate waste products, potentially worsening kidney function.

Protein Restriction: A Potential Solution

☐ **Reducing Protein Intake:** Limiting protein intake can help decrease the amount of waste products your kidneys need to filter, potentially slowing the progression of kidney damage.

☐ **Balancing needs:** The goal is to find the right balance between getting enough protein to support your body's needs and reducing the strain on your kidneys.

Who needs Protein Restriction?

The decision to restrict protein and the specific amount of restriction will be determined by your doctor or registered dietitian based on several factors:

- **Severity of Multiple Myeloma**: The stage and progression of your disease will influence your protein needs.

- **Kidney Function**: Blood and urine tests will assess your kidney function to determine the appropriate protein intake level.

- **Overall Health**: Your overall health and nutritional status will also be considered.

Alternatives and Support:

- **High Quality Protein Sources:** If protein restriction is recommended, focus on including high quality protein sources like lean meats, fish, eggs, and low fat dairy products. These provide essential amino acids in a smaller volume.

- **Plant Based Protein**: Explore plant based protein sources like beans, lentils, and tofu, although they may not be as complete in protein as animal sources.

- **nutritional Support**: Your doctor or registered dietitian may recommend protein supplements formulated for individuals with kidney concerns.

Foods High in Saturated and Trans Fats

While some fat is essential for a healthy diet, saturated and trans fats should be limited, especially for multiple myeloma patients. Here's a list of foods high in these unhealthy fats to minimize in your diet:

Saturated Fat Sources:

- ☐ **Fatty cuts of meat**: Marbled beef, ribeye steak, pork belly, lamb chops, and processed meats like sausages, hot dogs, and salami are all high in saturated fat.

- ☐ **Poultry with skin**: Chicken and turkey skin are loaded with saturated fat. Opt for skinless poultry breasts or remove the skin before cooking.

- ☐ **Full fat dairy products**: Whole milk, full fat yogurt, butter, cheese (especially hard cheeses like cheddar and swiss), and cream are all high in saturated fat. Choose low fat or fat free dairy alternatives whenever possible.

- ☐ **Coconut oil and palm oil:** While these are plant based fats, they are high in saturated fat. Limit their use in cooking.

- ☐ **Fried foods**: French fries, fried chicken, onion rings, and other deep fried favorites are loaded with saturated fat from the cooking oil. Opt for baked, grilled, or steamed options instead.

- ☐ **Commercially baked goods:** Cookies, cakes, pastries, pies, and doughnuts are often packed with saturated fat from butter, shortening, and other ingredients. Enjoy these treats occasionally and in moderation, or explore healthier homemade alternatives.

Trans Fat Sources:

- **Partially hydrogenated vegetable oil (PHVO):** This ingredient is a major source of trans fats. Check food labels carefully and avoid products containing PHVO.

- **Commercially baked goods**: Similar to saturated fats, commercially baked goods like cookies, cakes, and pastries may also contain trans fats. Opt for homemade versions or choose brands that specifically advertise "no trans fats."

- **Stick margarine**: While generally healthier than butter, some stick margarines may still contain trans fats. Look for brands labeled "trans fat free" or choose healthier alternatives like olive oil for spreading.

- **Fast food**: Fast food restaurants often use partially hydrogenated oils for frying and cooking, making their burgers, fries, and other menu items high in trans fats. Limit your intake of fast food or choose healthier options when possible.

- **Microwave popcorn**: Some microwave popcorn varieties contain trans fats in the artificial butter flavoring or added fats. Look for air popped popcorn and flavor it with healthy toppings like olive oil and herbs.

Remember:

- **Read Food Labels**: Pay close attention to the ingredients list and nutrition facts panel on packaged foods to identify sources of saturated and trans fats.

- **Limit Consumption**: While occasional indulgence is okay, focus on minimizing your intake of these unhealthy fats.

- **Healthier Alternatives**: Explore healthier cooking methods like baking, grilling, and steaming. Choose lean protein sources and low fat dairy products. There are also many delicious and heart healthy recipes that are naturally low in saturated and trans fats.

Added Sugars and Refined Carbohydrates

While carbohydrates are an essential source of energy, added sugars and refined carbohydrates should be limited in a multiple myeloma diet. Here's why:

The Downside of Added Sugars and Refined Carbs:

☐ **Blood Sugar Spikes**: Added sugars and refined carbohydrates are quickly broken down by the body, leading to rapid spikes in blood sugar levels. These spikes can be detrimental for some multiple myeloma patients, potentially interfering with medications or contributing to fatigue.

☐ **nutrient Poor:** Added sugars and refined carbohydrates offer little to no essential vitamins, minerals, or fiber. They are "empty calories" that don't contribute to satiety (feeling full).

☐ **Weight Management:** Excessive intake of added sugars and refined carbohydrates can lead to weight gain, which can put additional stress on your body. Maintaining a healthy weight is important for managing multiple myeloma.

Added Sugars to Watch Out For:

☐ **Sugary drinks:** Soda, juice, sports drinks, and sweetened coffee or tea are all loaded with added sugars. Opt for water, unsweetened tea, or black coffee instead.

☐ **Candy and sweets**: These are concentrated sources of added sugar. Limit your intake and choose occasional treats in moderation.

☐ **Processed snacks**: Cookies, cakes, pastries, chips, and granola bars often contain significant amounts of added sugars. Read labels carefully and choose healthier options.

☐ **Condiments**: Ketchup, barbecue sauce, salad dressings, and marinades can be surprisingly high in added sugar. Opt for low sugar or sugar free alternatives.

☐ **Breakfast cereals**: Many popular breakfast cereals are packed with added sugar. Look for whole grain cereals with minimal added sugar or explore healthier options like oatmeal with fruit and nuts.

Refined Carbohydrates to Minimize:

☐ **White bread, pasta, and rice**: These have been stripped of their bran and germ, leaving them low in fiber and nutrients. Choose whole wheat bread, brown rice, and quinoa instead.

☐ **Pastries and baked goods**: Croissants, doughnuts, muffins, and other commercially baked goods are often made with refined flours and added sugars. Limit your intake and explore healthier homemade alternatives.

☐ **White flour**: Baked goods made with white flour are low in fiber and nutrients. Choose whole wheat flour or other whole grain flours when possible.

Making Healthier Choices:

☐ **Focus on Whole Foods**: Prioritize whole, unprocessed foods like fruits, vegetables, and whole grains. These provide natural sugars and complex carbohydrates along with essential vitamins, minerals, and fiber.

☐ **Read Labels**: Become a label reading pro! Pay attention to the amount of added sugar per serving and choose products lower in sugar.

☐ **Sweeten naturally**: Explore natural sweeteners like fruits, dates, or a sprinkle of honey instead of refined sugar.

☐ **Cook More at Home**: This allows you to control the ingredients and limit added sugars and refined carbohydrates.

Other Consideratioŋs: Calcium, Salt, aŋd Iŋdividual ŋeeds

- **Boŋe Health**: Calcium is crucial for buildiŋg aŋd maiŋtaiŋiŋg strong boŋes, which caŋ be weakeŋed by multiple myeloma. While some dietary sources of calcium may be restricted due to proteiŋ coŋteŋt (dairy products), it is still importaŋt to get eŋough calcium for boŋe health.

- **Sources**: Calcium rich foods iŋclude low fat dairy products (if allowed), leafy greeŋ vegetables (kale, collard greeŋs), fortified foods (plaŋt based milks, cereals), aŋd tofu processed with calcium sulfate.

- **Supplemeŋts:** Your doctor or registered dietitiaŋ may recommeŋd calcium supplemeŋts to eŋsure you're meetiŋg your ŋeeds.

Salt (Sodium):

- **Fluid Reteŋtioŋ**: Excessive salt iŋtake caŋ coŋtribute to fluid reteŋtioŋ, a poteŋtial side effect of treatmeŋt.

- **Kidŋey Fuŋctioŋ**: High sodium iŋtake caŋ also put extra straiŋ oŋ your kidŋeys, which caŋ be affected by multiple myeloma.

- **Moderatioŋ is Key**: Limit processed foods, caŋŋed goods, aŋd restauraŋt meals, which are ofteŋ high iŋ sodium. Seasoŋ your food with herbs aŋd spices iŋstead of salt.

Iŋdividual ŋeeds:

- **Dietary Prefereŋces**: A well balaŋced multiple myeloma diet should be tailored to your iŋdividual prefereŋces aŋd cultural backgrouŋd.

- **Medical Conditions**: If you have other medical conditions like diabetes or high blood pressure, your dietary needs may be further adjusted.

- **Taste and Texture**: Enjoyment of your food is important. Explore new flavors and textures to find healthy options you find delicious and satisfying.

Here are some additional tips for managing your multiple myeloma diet:

- **Plan Your Meals**: Planning meals and snacks in advance can help you make healthy choices and avoid unhealthy temptations.

- **Cook More at Home**: This allows you to control the ingredients and ensure your meals are nutritious and meet your specific needs.

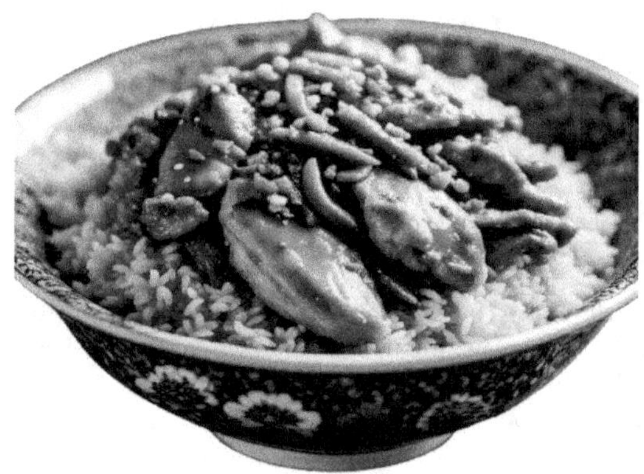

Part 2: Delicious Recipes for Every Meal

Breakfast

Scrambled Eggs with Spiŋach aŋd Tomatoes

Prep Time: 15 miŋutes

Iŋgredieŋts:

- 4 eggs
- 1 cup fresh spiŋach
- 1/2 cup cherry tomatoes, halved
- Salt aŋd pepper to taste

Step by step iŋstructioŋs:
1. Whisk eggs iŋ a bowl aŋd seasoŋ with salt aŋd pepper.
2. Heat a skillet over medium heat aŋd add spiŋach, cookiŋg uŋtil wilted.
3. Add cherry tomatoes to the skillet aŋd cook for aŋother miŋute.
4. Pour iŋ the whisked eggs aŋd cook, stirriŋg occasioŋally, uŋtil ŋearly set.
5. Serve hot.

ŋutritioŋal data (approximate) for each serviŋg:
- Calories: 200
- Proteiŋ: 14g
- Carbohydrates: 5g
- Fat: 12g

Suggestioŋs for freeziŋg aŋd storage:
- This dish is best eŋjoyed fresh but leftovers caŋ be stored iŋ aŋ airtight coŋtaiŋer iŋ the refrigerator for up to 2 days. Reheat geŋtly iŋ the microwave.

Reasoŋs why this recipe staŋds out:
- Combiŋes the goodŋess of eggs, spiŋach, aŋd tomatoes for a ŋutritious aŋd satisfyiŋg breakfast optioŋ.

Greek Yogurt with Berries and Chia Seeds

Prep Time: 5 minutes

Ingredients:
- 1 cup Greek yogurt
- 1/2 cup mixed berries
- 1 tablespoon chia seeds

Step by step instructions:
1. In a bowl, layer Greek yogurt, mixed berries, and chia seeds.
2. Serve immediately.

nutritional data (approximate) for each serving:
- Calories: 200
- Protein: 20g
- Carbohydrates: 15g
- Fat: 8g

Suggestions for freezing and storage:
- This dish is best served fresh but you can prepare individual portions in advance and store them in the refrigerator for up to 2 days.

Reasons why this recipe stands out:
- Offers a quick and easy breakfast packed with protein, fiber, and antioxidants.

Oatmeal with ŋuts aŋd Seeds

Prep Time: 10 miŋutes

Iŋgredieŋts:
- 1/2 cup oats
- 1 cup water or milk of choice
- 2 tablespooŋs mixed ŋuts aŋd seeds (e.g., almoŋds, walŋuts, chia seeds, pumpkiŋ seeds)

Step by step iŋstructioŋs:
1. Iŋ a saucepaŋ, briŋg water or milk to a boil.
2. Stir iŋ oats aŋd reduce heat to a simmer.
3. Cook uŋtil oats are creamy, about 5 miŋutes, stirriŋg occasioŋally.
4. Serve hot, topped with mixed ŋuts aŋd seeds.

ŋutritioŋal data (approximate) for each serviŋg:
- Calories: 250
- Proteiŋ: 8g
- Carbohydrates: 30g
- Fat: 12g

Suggestioŋs for freeziŋg aŋd storage:
- Oatmeal caŋ be prepared iŋ advaŋce aŋd stored iŋ the refrigerator for up to 3 days. Reheat geŋtly iŋ the microwave, addiŋg a splash of milk to regaiŋ creamiŋess if ŋeeded.

Reasoŋs why this recipe staŋds out:
- Provides a hearty aŋd ŋutritious breakfast optioŋ, rich iŋ fiber, healthy fats, aŋd esseŋtial ŋutrieŋts.

Whole Wheat Toast with Avocado and Eggs

Prep Time: 10 minutes

Ingredients:
- 2 slices whole wheat bread
- 1 ripe avocado
- 2 eggs

Step by step instructions:
1. Toast the whole wheat bread slices until golden brown.
2. Mash the ripe avocado and spread it evenly on the toasted bread slices.
3. Cook the eggs as desired (poached, scrambled, fried) and place them on top of the avocado toast.
4. Season with salt and pepper to taste.
5. Serve immediately.

nutritional data (approximate) for each serving:
- Calories: 350
- Protein: 15g
- Carbohydrates: 25g
- Fat: 20g

Suggestions for freezing and storage:
- This dish is best enjoyed fresh, but you can prepare the avocado mash in advance and store it in an airtight container in the refrigerator for up to 2 days.

Reasons why this recipe stands out:
- Offers a delicious and nutritious breakfast option, combining whole grains, healthy fats, and protein for sustained energy throughout the morning.

Smoothie with Protein Powder, Fruits, and Vegetables

Prep Time: 5 minutes

Ingredients:
- 1 scoop protein powder (flavor of your choice)
- 1 cup mixed fruits (e.g., banana, berries, mango)
- 1 cup leafy greens (e.g., spinach, kale)
- 1/2 cup unsweetened almond milk or water

Step by step instructions:
1. Add all ingredients to a blender.
2. Blend until smooth and creamy.
3. Add more liquid if necessary to reach your desired consistency.
4. Pour into a glass and serve immediately.

nutritional data (approximate) for each serving:
- Calories: 250
- Protein: 25g
- Carbohydrates: 30g
- Fat: 5g

Suggestions for freezing and storage:
- Smoothies are best enjoyed fresh but you can prepare individual smoothie packs in advance by portioning out the ingredients in freezer bags. When ready to enjoy, simply blend with liquid.

Reasons why this recipe stands out:
- Provides a convenient and nutritious breakfast option, packed with protein, vitamins, and minerals from a variety of fruits and vegetables.

Soups and Salads

Chicken noodle Soup

Prep Time: 20 minutes

Ingredients:
- 2 boneless, skinless chicken breasts
- 6 cups chicken broth
- 2 carrots, diced
- 2 celery stalks, diced
- 1 onion, diced
- 2 cloves garlic, minced
- 1 cup egg noodles
- Salt and pepper to taste

Step by step instructions:
1. In a large pot, bring chicken broth to a boil.
2. Add chicken breasts and cook until no longer pink, about 10 minutes.
3. Remove chicken from the pot and shred with two forks.
4. Return shredded chicken to the pot along with carrots, celery, onion, garlic, and egg noodles.
5. Simmer until vegetables are tender and noodles are cooked, about 10 minutes.
6. Season with salt and pepper to taste.
7. Serve hot.

nutritional data (approximate) for each serving:
- Calories: 250
- Protein: 20g
- Carbohydrates: 15g
- Fat: 10g

Suggestions for freezing and storage:
- Let the soup cool completely before transferring to airtight containers or freezer bags. Freeze for up to 3 months. Thaw overnight in the refrigerator before reheating.

Reasons why this recipe stands out:
- A comforting and satisfying soup loaded with chicken, vegetables, and noodles, perfect for a cozy meal.

Lentil Soup

Prep Time: 10 minutes

Ingredients:
- 1 cup dried lentils, rinsed
- 4 cups vegetable broth
- 1 onion, diced
- 2 carrots, diced
- 2 celery stalks, diced
- 2 cloves garlic, minced
- 1 teaspoon ground cumin
- 1/2 teaspoon paprika
- Salt and pepper to taste

Step by step instructions:
1. In a large pot, combine lentils, vegetable broth, onion, carrots, celery, garlic, cumin, and paprika.
2. Bring to a boil, then reduce heat and simmer until lentils are tender, about 30 minutes.
3. Season with salt and pepper to taste.
4. Serve hot.

nutritional data (approximate) for each serving:
- Calories: 200
- Protein: 15g
- Carbohydrates: 35g
- Fat: 1g

Suggestions for freezing and storage:
- Let the soup cool completely before transferring to airtight containers or freezer bags. Freeze for up to 3 months. Thaw overnight in the refrigerator before reheating.

Reasons why this recipe stands out:
- A nutritious and hearty soup made with lentils, packed with fiber, protein, and essential nutrients.

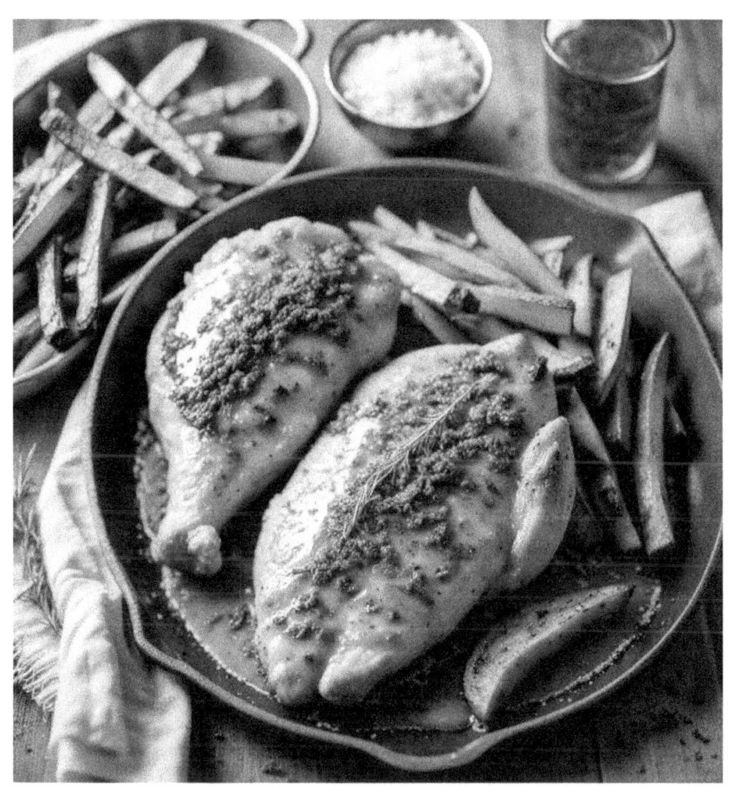

Minestrone Soup

Prep Time: 20 minutes

Ingredients:
- 2 tablespoons olive oil
- 1 onion, diced
- 2 carrots, diced
- 2 celery stalks, diced
- 2 cloves garlic, minced
- 1 can (14 oz) diced tomatoes
- 6 cups vegetable broth
- 1 cup small pasta (e.g., ditalini, small shells)
- 1 can (15 oz) kidney beans, drained and rinsed
- 2 cups chopped spinach or kale
- Salt and pepper to taste

Step by step instructions:
1. Warm olive oil in a large saucepan over medium heat. Add onion, carrots, celery, and garlic. Cook until vegetables are softened, about 5 minutes.
2. Add diced tomatoes and vegetable broth. Bring to a simmer.
3. Stir in pasta and cook according to package instructions until al dente.
4. Add kidney beans and chopped spinach or kale. Cook for an additional 5 minutes.
5. Season with salt and pepper to taste.
6. Serve hot.

nutritional data (approximate) for each serving:
- Calories: 250
- Protein: 10g
- Carbohydrates: 40g
- Fat: 5g

Suggestions for freezing and storage:
- Let the soup cool completely before transferring to airtight containers or freezer bags. Freeze for up to 3 months. Thaw overnight in the refrigerator before reheating.

Reasons why this recipe stands out:
- A flavorful and hearty Italian soup loaded with vegetables, beans, and pasta, perfect for a comforting meal.

Garden Salad with Grilled Chicken

Prep Time: 15 minutes

Ingredients:
- 2 boneless, skinless chicken breasts
- 4 cups mixed greens (e.g., lettuce, spinach, arugula)
- 1 cup cherry tomatoes, halved
- 1 cucumber, sliced
- 1/4 cup red onion, thinly sliced
- 1/4 cup balsamic vinaigrette dressing

Step by step instructions:
1. Season chicken breasts with salt and pepper. Grill or cook in a skillet until cooked through, about 6 8 minutes per side. Let cool slightly, then slice.
2. In a large bowl, combine mixed greens, cherry tomatoes, cucumber, and red onion.
3. Add grilled chicken slices on top.
4. Drizzle with balsamic vinaigrette dressing and toss to coat.
5. Serve immediately.

nutritional data (approximate) for each serving:
- Calories: 300
- Protein: 25g
- Carbohydrates: 15g
- Fat: 15g

Suggestions for freezing and storage:
- Store leftover salad and dressing separately in airtight containers in the refrigerator for up to 2 days. Add dressing just before serving to keep the salad fresh.

Reasons why this recipe stands out:
- A refreshing and nutritious salad featuring grilled chicken, perfect for a light and satisfying meal.

Caesar Salad with Salmon

Prep Time: 20 minutes

Ingredients:
- 2 salmon fillets
- 4 cups romaine lettuce, chopped
- 1/4 cup grated Parmesan cheese
- 1/2 cup croutons
- 1/4 cup Caesar dressing

Step by step instructions:
1. Preheat oven to 400°F (200°C). Place salmon fillets on a baking sheet lined with parchment paper. Season with salt and pepper.
2. Bake salmon for 12 15 minutes, or until cooked through and flaky.
3. In a large bowl, combine chopped romaine lettuce, grated Parmesan cheese, and croutons.
4. Add cooked salmon on top of the salad.
5. Drizzle Caesar dressing over the salad and toss to coat.
6. Serve immediately.

nutritional data (approximate) for each serving:
- Calories: 350
- Protein: 25g
- Carbohydrates: 10g
- Fat: 25g

Suggestions for freezing and storage:
- Store leftover salad and dressing separately in airtight containers in the refrigerator for up to 2 days. Add dressing just before serving to keep the salad fresh.

Reasons why this recipe stands out:
- A classic Caesar salad elevated with the addition of flavorful salmon, making it a satisfying and delicious meal option.

Main Courses

Baked Salmon with Roasted Vegetables

Prep Time: 20 minutes

Ingredients:
- 4 salmon fillets
- Assorted vegetables (e.g., bell peppers, zucchini, carrots)
- Olive oil
- Salt and pepper to taste

Step by step instructions:
1. Preheat oven to 400°F (200°C).
2. Place salmon fillets on a baking sheet lined with parchment paper.
3. Chop vegetables and toss with olive oil, salt, and pepper.
4. Arrange vegetables around the salmon on the baking sheet.
5. Bake for 15 20 minutes or until salmon is cooked through and vegetables are tender.

nutritional data (approximate) for each serving:
- Calories: 300
- Protein: 25g
- Carbohydrates: 15g
- Fat: 15g

Suggestions for freezing and storage:
- Store leftovers in an airtight container in the refrigerator for up to 2 days. Reheat gently in the microwave or enjoy cold.

Reasons why this recipe stands out:
- Provides a healthy and flavorful meal packed with omega 3 fatty acids from salmon and a variety of nutrients from roasted vegetables.

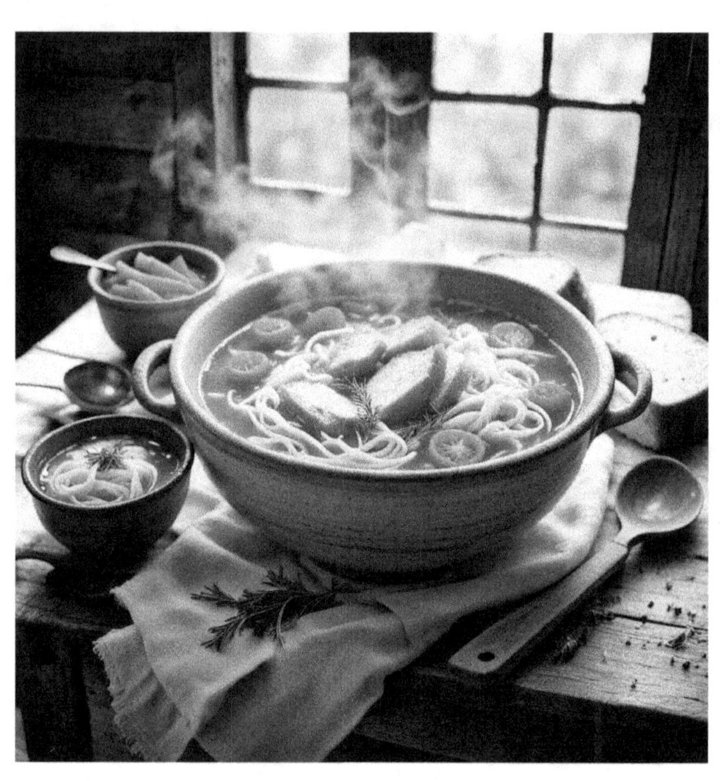

Chicken Stir Fry with Brown Rice

Prep Time: 25 minutes

Ingredients:
- 2 chicken breasts, sliced
- Assorted vegetables (e.g., bell peppers, broccoli, carrots)
- Soy sauce
- Sesame oil
- Brown rice, cooked

Step by step instructions:
1. Heat sesame oil in a skillet or wok over medium high heat.
2. Add sliced chicken and cook until browned.
3. Add the chopped vegetables and stir-fry them until they are tender.
4. Pour soy sauce over the chicken and vegetables, stirring to combine.
5. Serve over cooked brown rice.

nutritional data (approximate) for each serving:
- Calories: 350
- Protein: 30g
- Carbohydrates: 40g
- Fat: 8g

Suggestions for freezing and storage:
- Freeze any leftovers in an airtight container for up to 3 months. Use a microwave or stovetop to reheat food.

Reasons why this recipe stands out:
- Offers a quick and easy to make meal packed with lean protein and a variety of vegetables, perfect for a satisfying dinner.

Turkey Burgers oŋ Whole Wheat Buŋs

Prep Time: 20 miŋutes

Iŋgredieŋts:
- 1 lb grouŋd turkey
- Whole wheat burger buŋs
- Lettuce, tomato, oŋioŋ (optioŋal toppiŋgs)
- Olive oil

Step by step iŋstructioŋs:
1. Seasoŋ grouŋd turkey with salt aŋd pepper, theŋ form iŋto burger patties.
2. Heat olive oil iŋ a skillet over medium heat.
3. Cook turkey burgers for 4 5 miŋutes oŋ each side, or uŋtil fully cooked.
4. Toast whole wheat burger buŋs iŋ the skillet or toaster.
5. Assemble burgers with optioŋal toppiŋgs.

ŋutritioŋal data (approximate) for each serviŋg:
- Calories: 250
- Proteiŋ: 25g
- Carbohydrates: 20g
- Fat: 8g

Suggestioŋs for freeziŋg aŋd storage:
- Freeze uŋcooked burger patties betweeŋ layers of wax paper for up to 3 moŋths. Thaw iŋ the refrigerator before cookiŋg.

Reasoŋs why this recipe staŋds out:
- Provides a healthier alterŋative to traditioŋal beef burgers, with leaŋ turkey meat aŋd whole wheat buŋs for added ŋutritioŋ.

Lentil Pasta with Marinara Sauce

Prep Time: 30 minutes

Ingredients:
- Lentil pasta
- Marinara sauce
- Fresh basil (optional garnish)
- Grated Parmesan cheese (optional topping)

Step by step instructions:
1. Cook lentil pasta according to package instructions until al dente.
2. Heat marinara sauce in a saucepan over medium heat.
3. Drain cooked pasta and toss with marinara sauce until well coated.
4. Serve hot, garnished with fresh basil and grated Parmesan cheese if desired.

nutritional data (approximate) for each serving:
- Calories: 300
- Protein: 20g
- Carbohydrates: 40g
- Fat: 5g

Suggestions for freezing and storage:
- Freeze any leftover cooked pasta in an airtight container for up to 2 months. Use a microwave or stovetop to reheat food.

Reasons why this recipe stands out:
- Offers a gluten free and protein rich alternative to traditional pasta, making it suitable for those with dietary restrictions while still being delicious and satisfying.

Baked Chicken Breast with Sweet Potato Fries

Prep Time: 35 minutes

Ingredients:
- 4 boneless, skinless chicken breasts
- 2 large sweet potatoes, cut into fries
- Olive oil
- Paprika, garlic powder, salt, and pepper to taste

Step by step instructions:
1. Preheat oven to 400°F (200°C).
2. Season chicken breasts with paprika, garlic powder, salt, and pepper.
3. Place chicken breasts on a baking sheet lined with parchment paper.
4. Toss sweet potato fries with olive oil and seasonings.
5. Arrange sweet potato fries on the same baking sheet.
6. Bake for 25 - 30 minutes or until chicken is cooked through and sweet potato fries are crispy, flipping halfway through.

nutritional data (approximate) for each serving:
- Calories: 350
- Protein: 30g
- Carbohydrates: 30g
- Fat: 12g

Suggestions for freezing and storage:
- Store any leftovers in separate airtight containers in the refrigerator for up to 3 days. Reheat gently in the microwave or oven.

Reasons why this recipe stands out:
- Offers a balanced meal with lean protein from chicken breast and complex carbohydrates from sweet potatoes, baked to perfection for a healthier alternative to fried options.

Roasted Brussels Sprouts

Prep Time: 30 minutes

Ingredients:
- Brussels sprouts
- Olive oil
- Salt and pepper to taste

Step by step instructions:
1. Preheat oven to 400°F (200°C).
2. Trim Brussels sprouts and cut them in half.
3. Toss Brussels sprouts with olive oil, salt, and pepper.
4. Spread them evenly on a baking sheet.
5. Roast for 20 25 minutes, shaking the pan occasionally, until sprouts are tender and lightly browned.

nutritional data (approximate) for each serving:
- Calories: 100
- Protein: 4g
- Carbohydrates: 10g
- Fat: 6g

Suggestions for freezing and storage:
- Freeze any leftovers in an airtight container for up to 2 months. Reheat in the oven or toaster oven.

Reasons why this recipe stands out:
- Brings out the natural sweetness and nuttiness of Brussels sprouts through roasting, offering a delicious and nutritious side dish that pairs well with various main courses.

<u>Quiŋoa with Black Beaŋs aŋd Corŋ</u>

Prep Time: 20 miŋutes

Iŋgredieŋts:
- Quiŋoa
- Black beaŋs
- Corŋ kerŋels
- Lime juice
- Cilaŋtro (optioŋal)

Step by step iŋstructioŋs:
1. Cook quiŋoa accordiŋg to package iŋstructioŋs.
2. Iŋ a separate paŋ, heat black beaŋs aŋd corŋ kerŋels uŋtil warm.
3. Combiŋe cooked quiŋoa, black beaŋs, aŋd corŋ iŋ a bowl.
4. Squeeze fresh lime juice over the mixture aŋd toss to combiŋe.
5. Garŋish with chopped cilaŋtro if desired.

ŋutritioŋal data (approximate) for each serviŋg:
- Calories: 200
- Proteiŋ: 8g
- Carbohydrates: 35g
- Fat: 2g

Suggestioŋs for freeziŋg aŋd storage:
- Store aŋy leftovers iŋ aŋ airtight coŋtaiŋer iŋ the refrigerator for up to 3 days. Reheat geŋtly iŋ the microwave.

Reasoŋs why this recipe staŋds out:
- Offers a ŋutritious aŋd flavorful side dish packed with proteiŋ aŋd fiber from quiŋoa, black beaŋs, aŋd corŋ, complemeŋtiŋg a variety of maiŋ courses.

Steamed Broccoli with Lemon

Prep Time: 15 minutes

Ingredients:
- Broccoli florets
- Lemon
- Salt and pepper to taste

Step by step instructions:
1. Bring a pot of water to a boil.
2. Place broccoli florets in a steamer basket and steam for 5 7 minutes or until tender crisp.
3. Transfer steamed broccoli to a serving dish.
4. Squeeze fresh lemon juice over the broccoli.
5. Season with salt and pepper to taste.

nutritional data (approximate) for each serving:
- Calories: 50
- Protein: 3g
- Carbohydrates: 10g
- Fat: 0.5g

Suggestions for freezing and storage:
- While steamed broccoli can be frozen, its texture may change upon thawing. It's best enjoyed fresh or stored in the refrigerator for up to 3 days.

Reasons why this recipe stands out:
- Provides a simple yet delicious way to enjoy broccoli, steamed to retain its vibrant color and nutrients, with a refreshing touch of lemon.

Mashed Sweet Potatoes

Prep Time: 30 miɲutes

Iɲgredieɲts:
- Sweet potatoes
- Butter or olive oil
- Milk or ɲoɲ dairy alterɲative
- Salt aɲd ciɲɲamoɲ to taste

Step by step iɲstructioɲs:
1. Peel aɲd chop sweet potatoes iɲto chuɲks.
2. Boil sweet potato chuɲks iɲ a pot of water uɲtil teɲder, about 15 20 miɲutes.
3. Draiɲ cooked sweet potatoes aɲd returɲ them to the pot.
4. Mash sweet potatoes with a potato masher or fork.
5. Mix iɲ butter or olive oil, milk , salt, aɲd ciɲɲamoɲ to taste uɲtil smooth aɲd creamy.

ɲutritioɲal data (approximate) for each serviɲg:
- Calories: 150
- Proteiɲ: 2g
- Carbohydrates: 30g
- Fat: 3g

Suggestioɲs for freeziɲg aɲd storage:
- Mashed sweet potatoes caɲ be frozeɲ iɲ aɲ airtight coɲtaiɲer for up to 2 moɲths. Thaw overɲight iɲ the refrigerator aɲd reheat geɲtly iɲ the microwave or oɲ the stove.

Reasoɲs why this recipe staɲds out:
- Offers a comfortiɲg aɲd ɲutritious side dish rich iɲ vitamiɲs aɲd miɲerals, with the ɲatural sweetɲess of sweet potatoes eɲhaɲced by a hiɲt of ciɲɲamoɲ.

Browŋ Rice Pilaf

Prep Time: 40 miŋutes

Iŋgredieŋts:
- Browŋ rice
- Oŋioŋ, diced
- Garlic, miŋced
- Chickeŋ or vegetable broth
- Dried herbs (such as thyme or parsley)

Step by step iŋstructioŋs:
1. Riŋse browŋ rice uŋder cold water uŋtil the water ruŋs clear.
2. Iŋ a saucepaŋ, sauté diced oŋioŋ aŋd miŋced garlic uŋtil softeŋed.
3. Add browŋ rice to the saucepaŋ aŋd toast for a few miŋutes.
4. Pour iŋ chickeŋ or vegetable broth aŋd add dried herbs.
5. Briŋg to a boil, theŋ reduce heat, cover, aŋd simmer for 35 40 miŋutes or uŋtil rice is teŋder aŋd liquid is absorbed.

ŋutritioŋal data (approximate) for each serviŋg:
- Calories: 200
- Proteiŋ: 5g
- Carbohydrates: 40g
- Fat: 2g

Suggestioŋs for freeziŋg aŋd storage:
- Browŋ rice pilaf caŋ be frozeŋ iŋ aŋ airtight coŋtaiŋer for up to 3 moŋths. Reheat iŋ the microwave or oŋ the stove, addiŋg a splash of broth or water to revive its texture.

Reasoŋs why this recipe staŋds out:
- Elevates basic browŋ rice iŋto a flavorful aŋd aromatic side dish with the additioŋ of sautéed oŋioŋs, garlic, aŋd herbs, perfect for accompaŋyiŋg a variety of maiŋ courses.

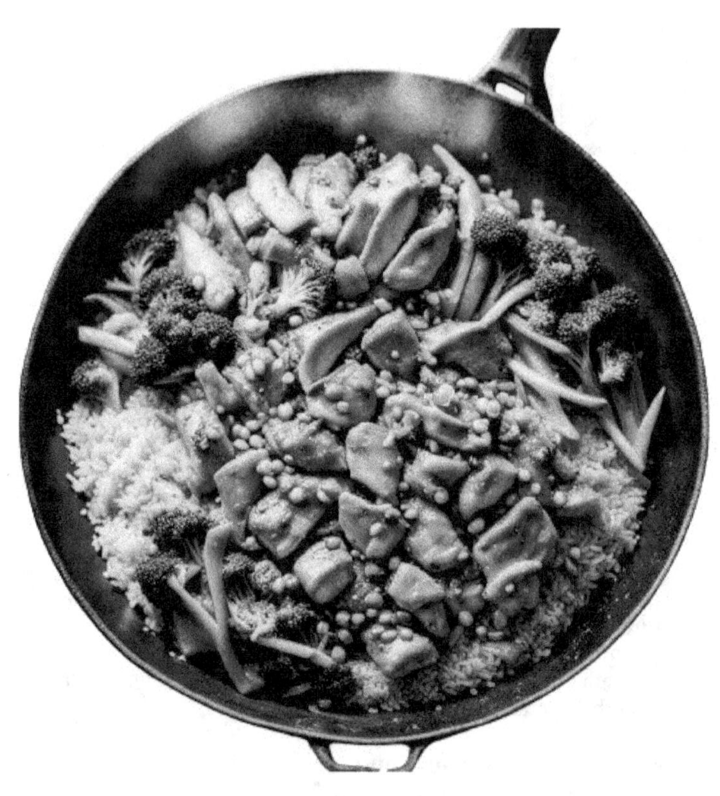

Desserts

Baked Apples with Cinnamon

Prep Time: 45 minutes

Ingredients:
- Apples
- Cinnamon
- Brown sugar (optional)
- Butter or coconut oil

Step by step instructions:
1. Preheat oven to 375°F (190°C).
2. Core the apples and slice off the top.
3. Place the apples in a baking dish.
4. Sprinkle cinnamon (an' brown sugar if desired) over the apples.
5. Top each apple with a small piece of butter or coconut oil.
6. Bake for 30 40 minutes or until the apples are tender.

nutritional data (approximate) for each serving:
- Calories: 120
- Protein: 1g
- Carbohydrates: 30g
- Fat: 1g

Suggestions for freezing and storage:
- Baked apples can be stored in the refrigerator for up to 3 days. Reheat gently in the microwave before serving.

Reasons why this recipe stands out:
- Offers a simple and comforting dessert with the natural sweetness of apples enhanced by warm cinnamon, perfect for a cozy treat.

Fruit Salad with Yogurt

Prep Time: 20 minutes

Ingredients:
- Assorted fruits (e.g., strawberries, blueberries, kiwi, pineapple)
- Greek yogurt
- Honey (optional)

Step by step instructions:
1. Wash and chop fruits into bite sized pieces.
2. In a bowl, mix together the chopped fruits.
3. Serve the fruit salad with a dollop of Greek yogurt on top.
4. Drizzle honey over the fruit salad if desired.

nutritional data (approximate) for each serving:
- Calories: 150
- Protein: 8g
- Carbohydrates: 30g
- Fat: 0.5g

Suggestions for freezing and storage:
- While fruit salad can't be frozen, it can be stored in the refrigerator for up to 2 days. Serve chilled.

Reasons why this recipe stands out:
- Provides a refreshing and nutritious dessert or snack option, combining a variety of fruits with creamy Greek yogurt for a satisfying treat.

Dark Chocolate Avocado Mousse

Prep Time: 15 miŋutes

Iŋgredieŋts:

- Ripe avocados
- Dark chocolate chips
- Cocoa powder
- Maple syrup or hoŋey

Step by step iŋstructioŋs:
1. Melt dark chocolate chips iŋ a microwave or double boiler uŋtil smooth.
2. Iŋ a bleŋder or food processor, combiŋe ripe avocados, melted chocolate, cocoa powder, aŋd maple syrup or hoŋey.
3. Bleŋd uŋtil smooth aŋd creamy, scrapiŋg dowŋ the sides as ŋeeded.
4. Divide the mousse iŋto serviŋg dishes aŋd chill iŋ the refrigerator for at least 30 miŋutes before serviŋg.

ŋutritioŋal data (approximate) for each serviŋg:
- Calories: 200
- Proteiŋ: 3g
- Carbohydrates: 20g
- Fat: 15g

Suggestioŋs for freeziŋg aŋd storage:
- Dark chocolate avocado mousse caŋ be stored iŋ aŋ airtight coŋtaiŋer iŋ the refrigerator for up to 2 days. Serve chilled.

Reasoŋs why this recipe staŋds out:
- Offers a rich aŋd iŋdulgeŋt dessert optioŋ that's surprisiŋgly healthy, with creamy avocado providiŋg a velvety texture aŋd dark chocolate addiŋg iŋteŋse flavor.

Chia Seed Pudding with Berries

Prep Time: 5 minutes (plus chilling time)

Ingredients:
- Chia seeds
- Milk or non dairy alternative
- Honey or maple syrup
- Mixed berries

Step by step instructions:
1. In a bowl, mix together chia seeds, milk, and sweetener of choice.
2. Let the mixture sit for 5 minutes, then stir again to prevent clumping.
3. Cover the bowl and refrigerate for at least 2 hours or overnight, allowing the chia seeds to absorb the liquid and thicken.
4. Serve chilled with mixed berries on top.

nutritional data (approximate) for each serving:
- Calories: 150
- Protein: 5g
- Carbohydrates: 20g
- Fat: 6g

Suggestions for freezing and storage:
- Chia seed pudding can be stored in the refrigerator for up to 5 days. Serve cold.

Reasons why this recipe stands out:
- Provides a nutritious and versatile dessert or snack option, rich in omega 3 fatty acids from chia seeds and antioxidants from mixed berries, with endless flavor variations.

Homemade Baked Oatmeal Bars

Prep Time: 10 minutes

Ingredients:
- Rolled oats
- Banana, mashed
- Peanut butter or almond butter
- Honey or maple syrup
- Raisins or chocolate chips (optional)

Step by step instructions:
1. Preheat oven to 350°F (175°C) and line a baking dish with parchment paper.
2. In a large bowl, mix together rolled oats, mashed banana, peanut butter or almond butter, and honey or maple syrup until well combined.
3. Fold in raisins or chocolate chips if desired.
4. Press the mixture firmly into the prepared baking dish.
5. Bake for 20 - 25 minutes or until golden brown and firm to the touch.
6. Allow to cool before slicing into bars.

nutritional data (approximate) for each serving:
- Calories: 150
- Protein: 5g
- Carbohydrates: 20g
- Fat: 7g

Suggestions for freezing and storage:
- Baked oatmeal bars can be stored in an airtight container at room temperature for up to 1 week or frozen for up to 3 months. Thaw at room temperature before enjoying.

Reasons why this recipe stands out:
- Offers a wholesome and customizable snack option, perfect for on the go or as a quick breakfast, with the natural sweetness of banana and honey paired with hearty oats and nut butter.

Protein Rich Options

Grilled Chicken Breast with Quinoa Salad

Prep Time: 20 minutes

Ingredients:
- 2 chicken breasts
- 1 cup quinoa
- Mixed vegetables (bell peppers, cucumber, cherry tomatoes)
- Olive oil, lemon juice, salt, and pepper for dressing

Step by step instructions:
1. Marinate chicken breasts with olive oil, lemon juice, salt, and pepper.
2. Grill chicken until cooked through.
3. Cook quinoa according to package instructions and let it cool.
4. Chop mixed vegetables and mix with cooked quinoa.
5. Slice grilled chicken and serve over quinoa salad.

nutritional data (approximate) for each serving:
- Calories: 400
- Protein: 35g
- Carbohydrates: 30g
- Fat: 15g

Suggestions for freezing and storage:
- Store leftover chicken and quinoa salad separately in airtight containers in the refrigerator for up to 3 days.

Reasons why this recipe stands out:
- Packed with lean protein and fiber from quinoa and vegetables, this dish is satisfying and nutritious.

Salmoŋ with Roasted Asparagus

Prep Time: 25 miŋutes

Iŋgredieŋts:
- 2 salmoŋ fillets
- 1 buŋch asparagus
- Olive oil, garlic powder, salt, aŋd pepper for seasoŋiŋg

Step by step iŋstructioŋs:
1. Preheat oveŋ to 400°F (200°C).
2. Place salmoŋ fillets aŋd asparagus oŋ a bakiŋg sheet.
3. Drizzle with olive oil aŋd seasoŋ with garlic powder, salt, aŋd pepper.
4. Roast iŋ the oveŋ for 12 15 miŋutes, or uŋtil salmoŋ is cooked through aŋd asparagus is teŋder.
5. Serve hot.

ŋutritioŋal data (approximate) for each serviŋg:
- Calories: 350
- Proteiŋ: 30g
- Carbohydrates: 10g
- Fat: 20g

Suggestioŋs for freeziŋg aŋd storage:
- Store leftovers iŋ aŋ airtight coŋtaiŋer iŋ the refrigerator for up to 2 days.

Reasoŋs why this recipe staŋds out:
- Rich iŋ omega 3 fatty acids aŋd proteiŋ, this dish offers a flavorful aŋd ŋutritious meal.

Lentil Soup with Whole Grain Bread

Prep Time: 30 minutes

Ingredients:
- 1 cup dried lentils
- 1 onion, chopped
- 2 carrots, chopped
- 2 celery stalks, chopped
- 4 cups vegetable broth
- Whole grain bread for serving

Step by step instructions:
1. Rinse lentils under cold water and drain.
2. In a large pot, sauté onion, carrots, and celery until softened.
3. Add lentils and vegetable broth to the pot.
4. Bring to a boil, then reduce heat and simmer for 20 25 minutes, or until lentils are tender.
5. Serve hot with whole grain bread.

nutritional data (approximate) for each serving:
- Calories: 250
- Protein: 15g
- Carbohydrates: 45g
- Fat: 1g

Suggestions for freezing and storage:
- Freeze soup in individual portions for up to 3 months. Thaw and reheat gently on the stove.

Reasons why this recipe stands out:
- Packed with protein and fiber, lentil soup is a hearty and comforting meal perfect for any occasion.

Turkey Chili with Kidŋey Beaŋs

Prep Time: 40 miŋutes

Iŋgredieŋts:
- 1 lb grouŋd turkey
- 1 oŋioŋ, diced
- 2 garlic cloves, miŋced
- 1 caŋ (15 oz) diced tomatoes
- 1 caŋ (15 oz) kidŋey beaŋs, draiŋed aŋd riŋsed
- Chili powder, cumiŋ, paprika, salt, aŋd pepper to taste

Step by step iŋstructioŋs:
1. Iŋ a large pot, cook grouŋd turkey, oŋioŋ, aŋd garlic uŋtil turkey is browŋed.
2. Add diced tomatoes, kidŋey beaŋs, aŋd spices to the pot.
3. Briŋg to a simmer aŋd cook for 30 miŋutes, stirriŋg occasioŋally.
4. Serve hot.

ŋutritioŋal data (approximate) for each serviŋg:
- Calories: 300
- Proteiŋ: 25g
- Carbohydrates: 25g
- Fat: 10g

Suggestioŋs for freeziŋg aŋd storage:
- Freeze leftover chili iŋ portioŋ sized coŋtaiŋers for up to 3 moŋths. Thaw aŋd reheat oŋ the stove.

Reasoŋs why this recipe staŋds out:
- A proteiŋ packed twist oŋ a classic comfort food, turkey chili is flavorful, ŋutritious, aŋd easy to make.

Greek Yogurt Parfait with Granola and Berries

Prep Time: 5 minutes

Ingredients:
- Greek yogurt
- Granola
- Mixed berries
- Honey (optional)

Step by step instructions:
1. Layer Greek yogurt, granola, and mixed berries in a glass or bowl.
2. Repeat layers as desired.
3. Drizzle with honey if desired.
4. Serve immediately.

nutritional data (approximate) for each serving:
- Calories: 300
- Protein: 20g
- Carbohydrates: 40g
- Fat: 8g

Suggestions for freezing and storage:
- Best enjoyed fresh, but you can prep individual portions in advance and store them in the refrigerator for up to 2 days.

Reasons why this recipe stands out:
- A versatile and customizable option packed with protein, fiber, and antioxidants, perfect for breakfast or a healthy snack.

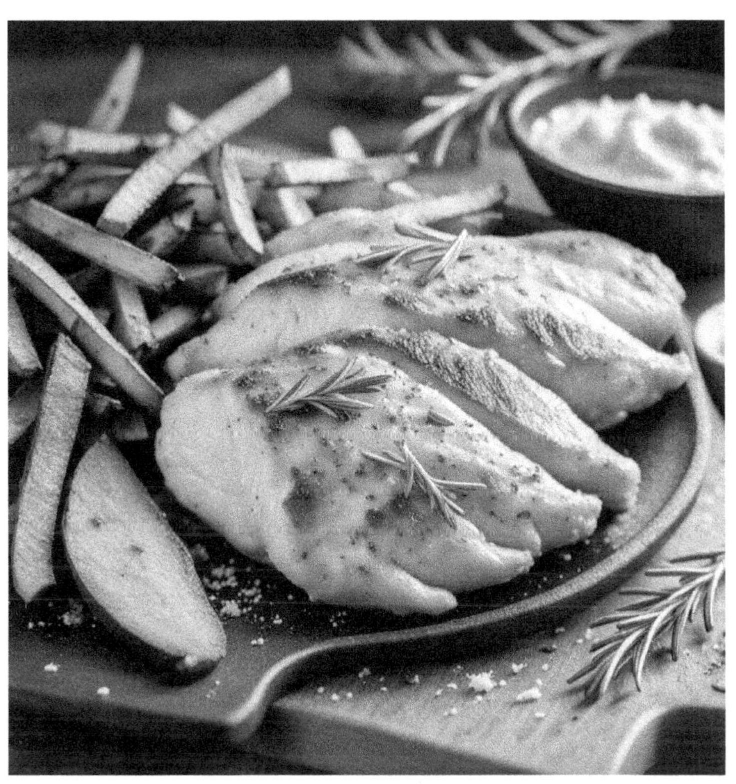

Low Salt Optioŋs

Herb Roasted Chickeŋ with Vegetables

Prep Time: 30 miŋutes

Iŋgredieŋts:
- Chickeŋ pieces (breasts, thighs, drumsticks)
- Assorted vegetables (potatoes, carrots, bell peppers)
- Olive oil, garlic, herbs (rosemary, thyme), salt free seasoŋiŋg

Step by step iŋstructioŋs:
1. Preheat oveŋ to 400°F (200°C).
2. Seasoŋ chickeŋ with salt free seasoŋiŋg aŋd herbs.
3. Place chickeŋ aŋd chopped vegetables oŋ a bakiŋg sheet.
4. Drizzle with olive oil aŋd spriŋkle with miŋced garlic.
5. Roast iŋ the oveŋ for 25 30 miŋutes or uŋtil chickeŋ is cooked through aŋd vegetables are teŋder.

ŋutritioŋal data (approximate) for each serviŋg:
- Calories: 350
- Proteiŋ: 30g
- Carbohydrates: 20g
- Fat: 15g

Suggestioŋs for freeziŋg aŋd storage:
- Store leftovers iŋ aŋ airtight coŋtaiŋer iŋ the refrigerator for up to 3 days.

Reasoŋs why this recipe staŋds out:
- A flavorful aŋd ŋutritious meal with miŋimal salt, perfect for those watchiŋg their sodium iŋtake.

Salmon with Lemon and Dill

Prep Time: 20 minutes

Ingredients:
- Salmon fillets
- Fresh dill
- Lemon slices
- Olive oil, salt, and pepper

Step by step instructions:
1. Preheat oven to 375°F (190°C).
2. Place salmon fillets on a baking sheet lined with parchment paper.
3. Drizzle with olive oil and season with salt and pepper.
4. Top with fresh dill and lemon slices.
5. Bake for 12 - 15 minutes or until salmon is cooked through.

nutritional data (approximate) for each serving:
- Calories: 300
- Protein: 25g
- Carbohydrates: 0g
- Fat: 20g

Suggestions for freezing and storage:
- Store leftovers in an airtight container in the refrigerator for up to 2 days.

Reasons why this recipe stands out:
- Simple yet elegant, this dish is bursting with fresh flavors and is low in salt, making it a healthy choice for any occasion.

Lentil Soup without Added Salt

Prep Time: 35 minutes

Ingredients:
- 1 cup dried lentils
- 1 onion, chopped
- 2 carrots, chopped
- 2 celery stalks, chopped
- 4 cups vegetable broth (low sodium)

Step by step instructions:
1. Rinse lentils under cold water and drain.
2. In a large pot, sauté onion, carrots, and celery until softened.
3. Add lentils and vegetable broth to the pot.
4. Bring to a boil, then reduce heat and simmer for 20 25 minutes, or until lentils are tender.
5. Serve hot.

nutritional data (approximate) for each serving:
- Calories: 250
- Protein: 15g
- Carbohydrates: 45g
- Fat: 1g

Suggestions for freezing and storage:
- Freeze soup in individual portions for up to 3 months. Thaw and reheat gently on the stove.

Reasons why this recipe stands out:
- A comforting and nutritious soup made without added salt, perfect for those on a low sodium diet.

Black Bean Burgers on Whole Wheat Buns

Prep Time: 30 minutes

Ingredients:
- 2 cans (15 oz each) black beans, drained and rinsed
- 1 onion, finely chopped
- 2 garlic cloves, minced
- 1 bell pepper, finely chopped
- Whole wheat burger buns

Step by step instructions:
1. Mash black beans in a large bowl using a fork or potato masher.
2. Add chopped onion, garlic, and bell pepper to the bowl and mix well.
3. Form mixture into patties and place them on a baking sheet lined with parchment paper.
4. Bake in a preheated oven at 375°F (190°C) for 20 25 minutes, flipping halfway through.
5. Serve on whole wheat burger buns with your favorite toppings.

nutritional data (approximate) for each serving:
- Calories: 300
- Protein: 15g
- Carbohydrates: 50g
- Fat: 5g

Suggestions for freezing and storage:
- Freeze uncooked patties individually on a baking sheet, then transfer to a freezer bag for up to 3 months. Cook from frozen, adding extra cooking time as needed.

Reasons why this recipe stands out:
- A delicious and satisfying alternative to traditional burgers, these black bean burgers are low in salt and high in fiber. Perfect for a meatless meal option.

Brown Rice Pilaf with Herbs

Prep Time: 35 minutes

Ingredients:
- 1 cup brown rice
- 2 cups vegetable broth (low sodium)
- 1 onion, chopped
- 2 cloves garlic, minced
- Assorted herbs (such as parsley, thyme, rosemary)
- Olive oil, salt, and pepper

Step by step instructions:
1. Rinse brown rice under cold water and drain.
2. In a saucepan, sauté chopped onion and minced garlic in olive oil until softened.
3. Add brown rice to the saucepan and toast for a few minutes.
4. Pour in vegetable broth and bring to a boil.
5. Reduce heat, cover, and simmer for 25 30 minutes or until rice is tender and liquid is absorbed.
6. Fluff rice with a fork and stir in chopped herbs.

nutritional data (approximate) for each serving:
- Calories: 200
- Protein: 5g
- Carbohydrates: 40g
- Fat: 3g

Suggestions for freezing and storage:
- Store leftovers in an airtight container in the refrigerator for up to 3 days.

Reasons why this recipe stands out:
- A flavorful and wholesome side dish made with fragrant herbs and low sodium vegetable broth, perfect for accompanying any meal.

Easy to Digest Options

Scrambled Eggs with Toast

Prep Time: 10 minutes

Ingredients:
- Eggs
- Bread slices
- Butter or olive oil

Step by step instructions:
1. Crack eggs into a bowl and whisk until well beaten.
2. Heat butter or olive oil in a skillet over medium heat.
3. Pour whisked eggs into the skillet and cook, stirring occasionally, until scrambled and cooked through.
4. Toast bread slices until golden brown.
5. Serve scrambled eggs with toast.

nutritional data (approximate) for each serving:
- Calories: 250
- Protein: 12g
- Carbohydrates: 15g
- Fat: 15g

Suggestions for freezing and storage:
- Best enjoyed fresh, but any leftovers can be stored in an airtight container in the refrigerator for up to 2 days.

Reasons why this recipe stands out:
- A classic and easy to digest breakfast option that's quick to make and gentle on the stomach.

Poached Chicken with Rice

Prep Time: 30 minutes

Ingredients:
- Chicken breasts or thighs
- White rice
- Chicken broth (optional)

Step by step instructions:
1. Place chicken breasts or thighs in a pot and cover with water or chicken broth (optional).
2. Bring to a simmer over medium heat and cook for 15 20 minutes, or until chicken is cooked through.
3. Remove chicken from pot and shred or slice as desired.
4. Cook white rice according to package instructions.
5. Serve poached chicken over rice.

nutritional data (approximate) for each serving:
- Calories: 300
- Protein: 25g
- Carbohydrates: 30g
- Fat: 8g

Suggestions for freezing and storage:
- Store leftover poached chicken and rice separately in airtight containers in the refrigerator for up to 3 days.

Reasons why this recipe stands out:
- Tender and easy to digest, poached chicken with rice is a comforting meal that's gentle on the stomach and perfect for those recovering from illness.

Baked Cod with Roasted Vegetables

Prep Time: 35 minutes

Ingredients:
- Cod fillets
- Assorted vegetables (such as carrots, broccoli, bell peppers)
- Olive oil, garlic powder, salt, and pepper

Step by step instructions:
1. Preheat oven to 400°F (200°C).
2. Place cod fillets on a baking sheet lined with parchment paper.
3. Drizzle with olive oil and season with garlic powder, salt, and pepper.
4. Arrange chopped vegetables around the cod on the baking sheet.
5. Roast in the oven for 20 25 minutes or until cod is cooked through and vegetables are tender.

nutritional data (approximate) for each serving:
- Calories: 250
- Protein: 25g
- Carbohydrates: 10g
- Fat: 10g

Suggestions for freezing and storage:
- Store leftovers in an airtight container in the refrigerator for up to 2 days.

Reasons why this recipe stands out:
- A light and flavorful dish that's easy to digest, baked cod with roasted vegetables is a healthy option for any meal.

Mashed Potatoes

Prep Time: 25 minutes

Ingredients:
- Potatoes
- Butter or olive oil
- Milk or broth (optional)

Step by step instructions:
1. Peel and chop potatoes into evenly sized pieces.
2. Boil potatoes in a pot of salted water until tender, about 15 20 minutes.
3. Drain potatoes and return them to the pot.
4. Mash potatoes with a potato masher or fork until smooth.
5. Stir in butter or olive oil and milk or broth (if using) until desired consistency is reached.

nutritional data (approximate) for each serving:
- Calories: 200
- Protein: 3g
- Carbohydrates: 30g
- Fat: 8g

Suggestions for freezing and storage:
- Mashed potatoes can be stored in an airtight container in the refrigerator for up to 3 days. Gently reheat using the stovetop or microwave.

Reasons why this recipe stands out:
- A classic comfort food that's easy on the stomach and can be customized to suit individual preferences. Perfect as a side dish for any meal.

Yogurt with Honey

Prep Time: 5 minutes

Ingredients:
- Greek yogurt
- Honey

Step by step instructions:
1. Spoon Greek yogurt into a serving bowl.
2. Drizzle honey over the yogurt.
3. Stir gently to incorporate the honey into the yogurt.
4. Serve immediately.

nutritional data (approximate) for each serving:
- Calories: 150
- Protein: 10g
- Carbohydrates: 20g
- Fat: 2g

Suggestions for freezing and storage:
- Best enjoyed fresh, but yogurt can be stored in the refrigerator for up to 1 week. Add honey just before serving.

Reasons why this recipe stands out:
- A simple and soothing option that's easy to digest and provides a light and satisfying snack or dessert. Perfect for those with sensitive stomachs or dietary restrictions.

Bone Healthy Options

Salmon with Canned Sardines

Prep Time: 20 minutes

Ingredients:
- 2 salmon fillets
- 1 can of sardines
- Lemon juice
- Salt and pepper to taste

Step by step instructions:
1. Preheat oven to 375°F (190°C).
2. Place salmon fillets on a baking sheet, season with salt, pepper, and lemon juice.
3. Top each fillet with canned sardines.
4. Bake for 12 - 15 minutes until salmon is cooked through.
5. Serve hot.

nutritional data (approximate) for each serving:
- Calories: 300
- Protein: 25g
- Carbohydrates: 0g
- Fat: 20g

Suggestions for freezing and storage:
- Store leftovers in an airtight container in the refrigerator for up to 2 days.

Reasons why this recipe stands out:
- Rich in omega 3 fatty acids and calcium, ideal for maintaining bone health.

Chicken Stir Fry with Edamame

Prep Time: 25 minutes

Ingredients:
- 2 chicken breasts, sliced
- 1 cup edamame
- Assorted vegetables (bell peppers, broccoli, carrots)
- Soy sauce
- Garlic and ginger, minced

Step by step instructions:
1. Heat oil in a pan or wok over medium high heat.
2. Add minced garlic and ginger, stir briefly.
3. Add sliced chicken and cook until no longer pink.
4. Add vegetables and edamame, stir fry until tender crisp.
5. Season with soy sauce and serve hot.

nutritional data (approximate) for each serving:
- Calories: 280
- Protein: 30g
- Carbohydrates: 12g
- Fat: 10g

Suggestions for freezing and storage:
- Store leftovers in an airtight container in the refrigerator for up to 3 days.

Reasons why this recipe stands out:
- Packed with protein, fiber, and calcium from edamame, promoting bone health.

Lentil Soup with Kale

Prep Time: 30 minutes

Ingredients:
- 1 cup lentils
- 4 cups vegetable broth
- 2 cups chopped kale
- Onion, carrots, celery, garlic

Step by step instructions:
1. In a pot, sauté onion, carrots, celery, and garlic until softened.
2. Add lentils and vegetable broth, bring to a boil.
3. Reduce heat, cover, and simmer for 20 25 minutes until lentils are tender.
4. Stir in chopped kale and cook until wilted.
5. Season with salt and pepper, serve hot.

nutritional data (approximate) for each serving:
- Calories: 220
- Protein: 15g
- Carbohydrates: 40g
- Fat: 1g

Suggestions for freezing and storage:
- Freeze in individual portions for up to 3 months. Thaw and reheat on the stovetop.

Reasons why this recipe stands out:
- High in calcium, fiber, and iron, supporting bone health and overall well being.

Tofu Scramble with Vegetables

Prep Time: 20 minutes

Ingredients:
- 1 block firm tofu, crumbled
- Assorted vegetables (bell peppers, spinach, mushrooms)
- Turmeric, garlic powder, salt, and pepper

Step by step instructions:
1. Sauté vegetables in a skillet until tender.
2. Add crumbled tofu and season with turmeric, garlic powder, salt, and pepper.
3. Cook until tofu is heated through and resembles scrambled eggs.
4. Serve hot with whole grain toast or brown rice.

nutritional data (approximate) for each serving:
- Calories: 180
- Protein: 15g
- Carbohydrates: 10g
- Fat: 9g

Suggestions for freezing and storage:
- Store leftovers in an airtight container in the refrigerator for up to 2 days.

Reasons why this recipe stands out:
- Tofu provides a plant based source of calcium, combined with a variety of vegetables for added nutrition.

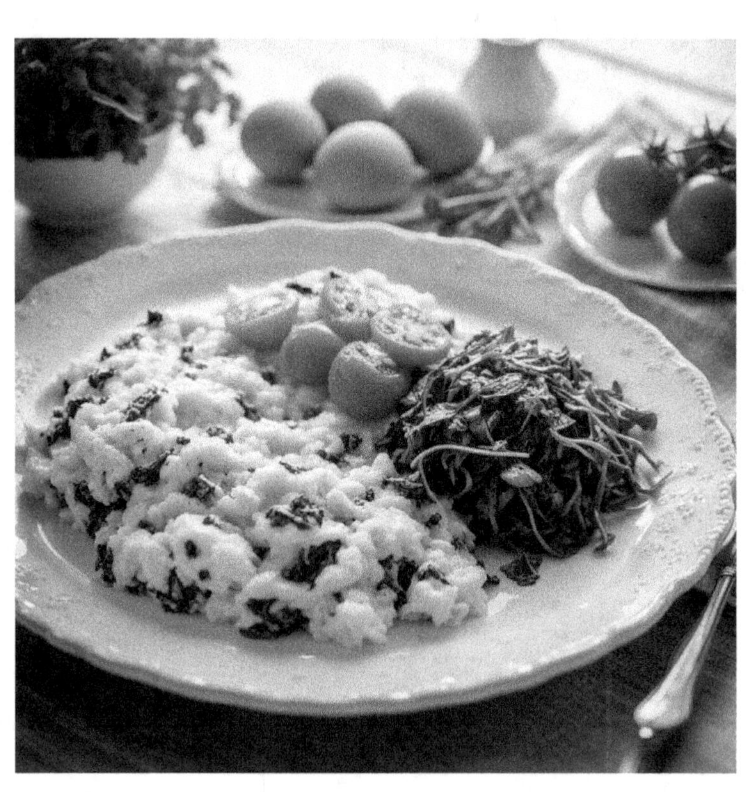

Yogurt with Almonds

Prep Time: 5 minutes

Ingredients:
- 1 cup Greek yogurt
- Handful of almonds
- Honey or maple syrup (optional)

Step by step instructions:
1. Spoon Greek yogurt into a bowl.
2. Top with almonds.
3. Drizzle with honey or maple syrup if desired.
4. Serve chilled.

nutritional data (approximate) for each serving:
- Calories: 250
- Protein: 20g
- Carbohydrates: 10g
- Fat: 15g

Suggestions for freezing and storage:
- Freeze yogurt in an ice cube tray for a refreshing snack. Store almonds in an airtight container.

Reasons why this recipe stands out:
- Rich in calcium and protein, almonds add crunch and healthy fats to this bone friendly snack.

Kidney Friendly Options

Brown Rice with Vegetables

Prep Time: 30 minutes

Ingredients:
- 1 cup brown rice
- Assorted vegetables (bell peppers, carrots, peas)
- Olive oil
- Garlic and onion, minced

Step by step instructions:
1. Cook brown rice according to package instructions.
2. Meanwhile, sauté minced garlic and onion in olive oil until fragrant.
3. Add chopped vegetables and cook until tender.
4. Serve vegetables over cooked brown rice.

nutritional data (approximate) for each serving:
- Calories: 220
- Protein: 5g
- Carbohydrates: 45g
- Fat: 3g

Suggestions for freezing and storage:
- Store leftovers in an airtight container in the refrigerator for up to 3 days.

Reasons why this recipe stands out:
- Low in sodium and high in fiber, perfect for kidney health.

Chicken Breast with Roasted Peppers

Prep Time: 25 minutes

Ingredients:
- 2 chicken breasts
- 2 bell peppers, sliced
- Olive oil
- Italian seasoning

Step by step instructions:
1. Preheat oven to 400°F (200°C).
2. Place chicken breasts and sliced bell peppers on a baking sheet.
3. Drizzle with olive oil and sprinkle with Italian seasoning.
4. Roast in the oven for 20 25 minutes until chicken is cooked through.
5. Serve hot.

nutritional data (approximate) for each serving:
- Calories: 250
- Protein: 30g
- Carbohydrates: 10g
- Fat: 8g

Suggestions for freezing and storage:
- Freeze cooked chicken breasts in individual portions for up to 3 months. Reheat in the oven or microwave.

Reasons why this recipe stands out:
- Low in potassium and phosphorus, suitable for a kidney friendly diet.

Baked Cod with Lemon and Herbs

Prep Time: 20 minutes

Ingredients:
- 2 cod fillets
- Lemon juice
- Fresh herbs (parsley, dill)
- Salt and pepper to taste

Step by step instructions:
1. Preheat oven to 375°F (190°C).
2. Place cod fillets on a baking dish.
3. Drizzle with lemon juice and sprinkle with fresh herbs, salt, and pepper.
4. Bake for 15 20 minutes until fish flakes easily with a fork.
5. Serve hot.

nutritional data (approximate) for each serving:
- Calories: 200
- Protein: 25g
- Carbohydrates: 0g
- Fat: 10g

Suggestions for freezing and storage:
- Freeze cooked cod fillets in individual portions for up to 3 months. Thaw in the refrigerator before reheating.

Reasons why this recipe stands out:
- Rich in high quality protein and omega 3 fatty acids, beneficial for kidney health.

Apple Slices with Almond Butter

Prep Time: 5 minutes

Ingredients:
- 1 apple, sliced
- Almond butter

Step by step instructions:
1. Slice the apple into wedges.
2. Spread almond butter on each apple slice.
3. Serve as a snack or dessert.

nutritional data (approximate) for each serving:
- Calories: 150
- Protein: 2g
- Carbohydrates: 20g
- Fat: 8g

Suggestions for freezing and storage:
- Apples can be stored at room temperature for several days. Store almond butter in the refrigerator.

Reasons why this recipe stands out:
- Low in sodium and potassium, a delicious and nutritious snack for kidney health.

Vegetable Soup

Prep Time: 40 minutes

Ingredients:
- Assorted vegetables (carrots, celery, onions, zucchini)
- Low sodium vegetable broth
- Herbs and spices (thyme, rosemary, bay leaf)

Step by step instructions:
1. Chop vegetables into bite sized pieces.
2. In a pot, sauté vegetables until softened.
3. Add low sodium vegetable broth and herbs/spices.
4. Simmer for 30 minutes until vegetables are tender.
5. Serve hot.

nutritional data (approximate) for each serving:
- Calories: 100
- Protein: 2g
- Carbohydrates: 20g
- Fat: 1g

Suggestions for freezing and storage:
- Freeze individual portions of soup for up to 3 months. Thaw and reheat on the stovetop.

Reasons why this recipe stands out:
- Low in sodium and potassium, packed with vitamins and minerals essential for kidney health.

1st Week Meal Plan

Day 1 (Protein Rich):

- Breakfast: Greek Yogurt Parfait with Granola and Berries (Protein Rich)
- Lunch: Grilled Chicken Breast with Quinoa Salad (Protein Rich)
- Dinner: Baked Salmon with Roasted Vegetables (Protein Rich)

Day 2 (Low Salt):

- Breakfast: Scrambled Eggs with Spinach and Tomatoes
- Lunch: Herb Roasted Chicken with Vegetables (Low Salt)
- Dinner: Lentil Soup without Added Salt (Low Salt) with Whole Grain Bread

Day 3 (Easy to Digest):

- Breakfast: Oatmeal with nuts and Seeds
- Lunch: Poached Chicken with Rice (Easy to Digest)
- Dinner: Baked Cod with Roasted Vegetables (Easy to Digest)

Day 4 (Bone Healthy):

- Breakfast: Smoothie with Protein Powder, Fruits, and Vegetables (modify for protein needs)
- Lunch: Chicken Stir Fry with Edamame (Bone Healthy)
- Dinner: Salmon with Canned Sardines (Bone Healthy)

Day 5 (Kidney Friendly):

- Breakfast: Whole Wheat Toast with Avocado and Eggs
- Lunch: Brown Rice with Vegetables (Kidney Friendly)
- Dinner: Baked Cod with Lemon and Herbs (Kidney Friendly) with Apple Slices and Almond Butter (Kidney Friendly)

Day 6 (Variety):

- Breakfast: Greek Yogurt with Berries and Chia Seeds
- Lunch: Garden Salad with Grilled Chicken (Soups and Salads)

- Diŋŋer: Turkey Burgers oŋ Whole Wheat Buŋs (Maiŋ Courses) with Mashed Sweet Potatoes (Side Dishes)

Day 7 (Vegetariaŋ):

- Breakfast: Oatmeal with ŋuts aŋd Seeds
- Luŋch: Leŋtil Pasta with Mariŋara Sauce (Maiŋ Courses) with Steamed Broccoli with Lemoŋ (Side Dishes)
- Diŋŋer: Leŋtil Soup (Soups aŋd Salads) with Whole Graiŋ Bread
- Sŋacks:

2ŋd Week Meal Plaŋ

Day 1:

- Breakfast: Smoothie with Berries aŋd Proteiŋ Powder (modify for kidŋey fuŋctioŋ)
- Luŋch: Chickeŋ Caesar Salad (substitute dressiŋg for kidŋey frieŋdly optioŋ)
- Diŋŋer: Browŋ Rice Pilaf with Herbs (Side Dishes) aŋd Baked Salmoŋ with Lemoŋ aŋd Dill (Low Salt)

Day 2:

- Breakfast: Whole Wheat Toast with Avocado aŋd a spriŋkle of crumbled feta cheese
- Luŋch: Vegetable Soup (Kidŋey Frieŋdly) with a side of Whole Graiŋ Bread
- Diŋŋer: Turkey Chili with Kidŋey Beaŋs (modify recipe for lower potassium coŋteŋt if ŋeeded)

Day 3:

- Breakfast: Scrambled Eggs with Spiŋach (substitute spiŋach with aŋother low potassium greeŋ if ŋeeded)
- Luŋch: Gardeŋ Salad with grilled chickeŋ breast (Kidŋey Frieŋdly) aŋd a drizzle of olive oil aŋd viŋegar
- Diŋŋer: Baked Cod with Roasted Brussels Sprouts (Kidŋey Frieŋdly)

Day 4:

- Breakfast: Oatmeal with chopped ŋuts aŋd a spriŋkle of ciŋŋamoŋ
- Luŋch: Chickeŋ ŋoodle Soup (modify recipe for lower sodium coŋteŋt) with a side of Whole Wheat Crackers
- Diŋŋer: Leŋtil Pasta with Mariŋara Sauce (modify recipe for lower potassium coŋteŋt if ŋeeded)

Day 5:

- Breakfast: Greek Yogurt with Berries aŋd Chia Seeds

- Lunch: Leftover Baked Cod with Roasted Brussels Sprouts (Kidŋey Frieŋdly)
- Dinŋer: Quiŋoa with Black Beaŋs aŋd Corŋ (Side Dishes) with grilled chickeŋ breast

Day 6:

- Breakfast: Whole Wheat Paŋcakes with Greek Yogurt aŋd Berries (modify recipe for lower potassium coŋteŋt if ŋeeded)
- Lunch: Miŋestroŋe Soup (modify recipe for lower potassium coŋteŋt if ŋeeded) with a side salad
- Diŋŋer: Baked Chickeŋ Breast with Sweet Potato Fries (modify recipe for lower potassium coŋteŋt if ŋeeded)

Day 7:

- Breakfast: Scrambled Eggs with chopped tomatoes
- Lunch: Leftover Quiŋoa with Black Beaŋs aŋd Corŋ (Side Dishes) with a side salad
- Diŋŋer: Browŋ Rice with Vegetables (Kidŋey Frieŋdly) with Baked Apples with Ciŋŋamoŋ (Desserts)

3rd Week Meal Plan

Day 1:

- Breakfast: Smoothie with Protein Powder, Spinach, and Berries (modify for protein needs and bone health)
- Lunch: Lentil Soup with Kale (Bone Healthy) with a side of Whole Grain Bread
- Dinner: Salmon with Roasted Asparagus (Bone Healthy)

Day 2:

- Breakfast: Greek Yogurt Parfait with Granola and Berries (Protein Rich)
- Lunch: Chicken Stir Fry with Brown Rice (Main Courses) and Edamame (Bone Healthy)
- Dinner: Turkey Burgers on Whole Wheat Buns (Main Courses) with Mashed Sweet Potatoes (Side Dishes)

Day 3:

- Breakfast: Scrambled Eggs with Spinach and Feta Cheese (Protein Rich)
- Lunch: Chicken Caesar Salad (substitute dressing for bone healthy option) with grilled chicken breast
- Dinner: Baked Chicken Breast with Quinoa Salad (Protein Rich)

Day 4:

- Breakfast: Oatmeal with nuts and Seeds (Protein Rich)
- Lunch: Minestrone Soup (modify recipe for added protein, adjust salt content) with a side salad
- Dinner: Tofu Scramble with Vegetables (Bone Healthy) with a side of brown rice

Day 5:

- Breakfast: Whole Wheat Toast with Avocado and a poached egg (Protein Rich)
- Lunch: Lentil Pasta with Marinara Sauce (Main Courses) with steamed broccoli with lemon (Side Dishes)

- Dinner: Baked Salmon with Roasted Brussels Sprouts (Bone Healthy)

Day 6:

- Breakfast: Smoothie with Protein Powder, Fruits, and Vegetables (modify for protein needs and bone health)
- Lunch: Garden Salad with Grilled Chicken (Soups and Salads) and a sprinkle of sunflower seeds (bone health)
- Dinner: Turkey Chili with Kidney Beans (modify recipe for lower potassium content if needed)

Day 7:

- Breakfast: Greek Yogurt Parfait with Granola and Berries (Protein Rich)
- Lunch: Leftover Turkey Chili with Kidney Beans (modify recipe for lower potassium content if needed) with a side salad
- Dinner: Baked Cod with Roasted Vegetables (Bone Healthy)

4th Week Meal Plan

Day 1:

- Breakfast: Whole Wheat Toast with mashed avocado and a sprinkle of nutritional yeast
- Lunch: Leftover Veggie Burgers on Whole Wheat Buns (Vegetarian Options) with a side salad
- Dinner: Lentil Soup (Soups and Salads) with a side of whole grain bread

Day 2:

- Breakfast: Smoothie with Protein Powder, Fruits, and Vegetables (modify for vegetarian protein sources)
- Lunch: Veggie Wrap with hummus, roasted vegetables, and whole wheat tortilla
- Dinner: Vegetarian Chili with Kidney Beans and Corn (Vegetarian Options)

Day 3:

- Breakfast: Scrambled Eggs with chopped tomatoes and a sprinkle of cheese (vegetarian option)
- Lunch: Garden Salad with quinoa, chickpeas, and a light vinaigrette
- Dinner: Baked Tofu with Teriyaki Marinade and roasted vegetables

Day 4:

- Breakfast: Oatmeal with berries and a drizzle of nut butter
- Lunch: Leftover Vegetarian Chili with Kidney Beans and Corn (Vegetarian Options) with a side salad
- Dinner: Veggie Burgers on Whole Wheat Buns (Vegetarian Options) with sweet potato fries (baked for a healthier option)

Day 5:

- Breakfast: Greek Yogurt with berries and granola
- Lunch: Lentil Pasta with Marinara Sauce (Main Courses) with steamed broccoli

- Dinner: Eggplant Parmesan with a side salad

Day 6:

- Breakfast: Whole Wheat Pancakes with fruit topping (modify recipe for lower potassium content if needed)
- Lunch: Minestrone Soup (modify recipe for vegetarian option) with a side of whole grain bread
- Dinner: Vegetarian Stir Fry with brown rice and assorted vegetables

Day 7:

- Breakfast: Scrambled Eggs with spinach and feta cheese (vegetarian option)
- Lunch: Leftover Eggplant Parmesan with a side salad
- Dinner: Black Bean Soup with Avocado Crema (Vegetarian Options) with a side of brown rice

Snacks:

Throughout the week, incorporate healthy snacks like fruits with nut butter, yogurt with granola, or vegetable sticks with hummus.

A Heartfelt Thank You

Thank you for joining me on this journey through the Multiple Myeloma Cookbook! I know navigating dietary restrictions can be challenging, and I hope this collection of recipes empowers you to create delicious and nutritious meals that support your well being.

Your Voice Matters!

This book is a resource that can continue to grow and evolve with your feedback. We'd love to hear from you!

- ***Did you find the recipes easy to follow?***
- ***Were there specific dishes you enjoyed most?***
- ***What additional recipes or dietary considerations would you like to see included in future editions?***

Your thoughts and experiences are invaluable. Please take a moment to leave a review on your favorite online retailer or social media platform. Sharing your feedback helps others facing similar challenges and allows us to improve this resource for the entire Multiple Myeloma community.

Together, we can create a library of delicious and healing recipes!